Birthing

Choices You Have to Create the Best Birth Experience for You and Your Baby

by
Irene Byrne, MA

Regula Burki, MD, FACOG, Medical Editor

Kim H. Burgess, BS, Editor

pince-nez press
san francisco

Birthing: Choices You Have to Create the Best Birth Experience For You and Your Baby
© 2003 Pince-Nez Press
All rights reserved.
Printed in the U.S.A.
ISBN 1-930074-06-9
Library of Congress Catalog Card No. 2002112494

Cover design page design & layout: Idintdoit Design
Fonts: Janson Text, Avant Garde, Bikley Script LET

Legal disclaimer: The information contained in this guide is intended not as medical advice; rather it is intended to direct readers to the birth professionals who can answer their medical questions specific to their personal situations and advise them on how they can best achieve a healthy delivery. All of the information in this book constitutes opinions of the contributing authors who are advocating for their preferred birth methods. Readers need to assess these opinions in conjunction with a birth professional who is aware of the reader's own personal situation and physical condition as well as their baby's, so they can make informed decisions that will best lead to the birth of a healthy baby.

This book is not a comprehensive guide to pregnancy and it does not address necessary prenatal care. Pregnant women need to seek this information elsewhere, as well as information on the warning signs that a pregnancy may be in trouble.

Pince-Nez Press
San Francisco, CA
(415) 267-5978 fax (800) 579-3614
www.pince-nez.com
info@pince-nez.com

Contents

Introduction: The Birth of a Book — 7

PART ONE: Giving Birth — 9
Birth Experiences — 10
Birth Statistics and Facts — 40
Questions to Ask in Planning Your Baby's Birth — 44

PART TWO: Choices of Birth Professionals — 49
Physicians — 50
Midwives — 57
Doulas — 76

PART THREE: Choices of Birth Techniques — 81
Lamaze — 84
The Bradley Method — 88
Waterbirth — 90
Hypnobirth — 97

PART FOUR: Choices of Where to Give Birth — 101
Hospitals — 102
Birthing Centers — 103
Home Births — 105

PART FIVE: Choices Regarding Interventions — 113
Induction — 114
Drugs to Induce Labor — 115

Other Methods of Inducing Labor	115
Labor Pain	116
Spinal Nerve Block	117
Epidural Nerve Block	117
Combined Spinal Block/Epidural Block	117
Fetal Monitoring	118
Episiotomy	119
Forceps/Vacuum Extraction	120
C-Section	121
PART SIX: Choices of the Birth Environment and Managing Labor	133
Who Present	134
Handling Inquiries	134
What Props	135
Birthing Positions	135
Birth Balls	139
Relaxation and Childbirth	143
Coping with Labor	144
Pregnancy and Labor Guidelines	147
PART SEVEN: Choices Regarding the Moment of Birth	153
After the Baby is Born	154
Taking Care of the Newborn	157
Taking Care of the New Mom	159
Breast-feeding	160

PART EIGHT: Birth Customs Around the World	171
PART NINE: Birth Plans	183
Birth Plan Statistics	184
Birth Plan Worksheet	189
Writing Your Birth Plan	193
Your Birth Plan	194
Irene's Birth Plan	197
PART TEN: Preparing for the Birth	199
Prenatal Care	200
Preparing Your Labor Team	210
What To Bring To The Hospital	211
What You Will Need at Home	211
PART ELEVEN: Prenatal Fun	213
A First Day Project: A Birth Day Memory Box	214
A Prenatal Project: Belly Casting	215
Acronyms	218
Index	219

Contributing authors and organizations

(alphabetical)

AUTHORS
17 moms and partners describing 20 birth experiences
Connie Banack, CD
Regula E. Burki, MD, FACOG
Jill Cohen, Midwife
Marci O'Daffer, CCE, Doula
Barbara Harper, RN
Sheila Kitzinger
Jack Newman, MD, FRCPC
Jennifer Normoyle, MD, OB/GYN
Mary Paliescheskey, BS
Paulina G. Perez, RN, BSN, FACCE, CD
Nancy Sullivan, CNM, MS, FACNM
Julie Tupler, RN
Kerry Tuschhoff, HBCE

ORGANIZATIONS
American Academy of Husband-Coached Childbirth
Coalition for Improving Maternity Services
Doulas of North America (DONA)
International Cesarean Awareness Network
International Childbirth Education Association
La Leche League International
Lamaze International
Midwifery Today
Midwives' Alliance of North America
Mothering the Mother Newsletter
National Center for Health Statistics

Introduction

The need for this book arose from the realization that childbirth itself has gone through a "rebirth" over the past ten years. Women now have many more birth options than before. The selection of a birthing environment is the first decision to be made. Women can choose to give birth at home, at the hospital or at a birthing center. In conjunction with this comes the decision of the type of assistance one may want at the birth. Apart from one's partner or coach, it is possible to have a physician, midwife, doula and/or a labor nurse to provide additional support. There is also the factor of medication or the choice of a "natural birth." The possible details are endless.

Over the course of their pregnancies, many women create birth plans detailing the choices they have made regarding the birth. Whether one actually lays out step by step each part of the birth plan varies from person to person. However, it is becoming increasingly common for women to enter into the final stages of their pregnancy with a written birth plan in hand. Of course, a birth plan is only a plan! It is important to remember that at the actual time of birth not all the details may go as expected. At the end of the day, the most important goal is a healthy mom and baby. This book includes a sample birth plan that you can use to plan for your baby's birth.

The preparation for the birth of a baby has really become a research project. This book is an attempt to present all the options that are currently available. This information is a compilation of articles from web sites, articles specifically written for this book and information in other childbirth books. All sources are listed. Also presented is information on the history of birthing customs and the way that tradition and culture may have influenced current birthing trends. The book includes testimonials from moms and partners about their birth experiences; guidelines and tips about labor, delivery, and birth; and general information about health and fitness during pregnancy. A section on breast-feeding is also included, since after labor and delivery it is the most important skill that a new mother may need. In the end, birth remains both a miracle and to some extent a mystery. We can plan and prepare all we want, but each birth will unfold in its own unique way.

Irene Byrne, MA

Dedication

To my husband, Tim, and our two beautiful children, Cliodhna and Carrig.

Special Acknowledgment

Thank you to Phuong Le for all her hard work on this project. It would never have been completed without her efficient help.

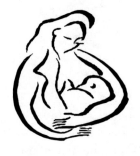

Part One: Giving Birth

Birth Experiences

Childbirth is full of surprises, as you can see from the testimonials below. Yes, go ahead and plan, but be flexible and prepared for whatever might happen. One mother commented, "The birth plan didn't make it out of my bag." Remember, this is about having a successful birth—meaning a healthy baby. You may have to put aside your personal desires to achieve this ultimate goal. Read below what other parents expected and what actually happened. Being flexible and open to surprises will prepare you well for your role as a parent!

If some of the terms used by the writers are unfamiliar, please refer to the index at the back of this book, which will direct you to definitions.

MIRACLE AND WONDER OF LIFE

The birth of my son, Aaron, began at my appointment at Dr. Miller's office in the morning. Dr. Miller checked to see how I was progressing and since I was a week overdue, she helped things along by pressing on my cervix. When I saw the blood, I knew the labor would start soon. I was excited, but tried to remain calm. At home, I rested on the couch most of the afternoon feeling minor, period-like cramps. By 7 p.m., the contractions had grown in strength and regularity enough that my husband, Dwight, and I began to keep track of them on paper. The frequency of the contractions and their intensity increased steadily. The contractions reminded me of the terrible and frightening period cramps that I had when I first started menstruating, but, because they were familiar, they were not so terrible or frightening now. I practiced breathing, trying to focus on making the first breath a welcoming one and trying to relax my body as best I could.

By 11 p.m., the contractions were quite strong and I was bleeding a lot. I had diarrhea, which cleared out my system but didn't make me feel very good. Dwight called the labor and delivery department at the hospital primarily out of concern for the blood loss, and they told us to come in as soon as we wanted. I preferred to spend as much time as possible at home where things were familiar and comfortable, so we waited another hour and a half before gathering our things and calling my sister, Barbara. We'd been listening to Isaac Hayes on the stereo, and I'd found it so soothing that I wouldn't let Dwight turn it off until just before we walked out the door.

When we got in the car, the time was 12:34 a.m. We immediately put on the Isaac Hayes CD. Since it was the middle of the night, there were few cars out and we made good time with a lot of green lights greeting our way. Dwight dropped me off at the emergency room and went to park the car, leaving me alone for what felt like half an hour. To get to the labor and delivery department, you have to walk a long maze of corridors, which, fortunately, have handrails along the way. Within minutes of getting settled into our room, Barbara arrived. My contractions were coming every three minutes and lasting about 30-40 seconds at a time. I was monitored for a while, and then allowed to move freely about our room.

Dwight and Barbara were wonderful. They said and did all the right things. I kept them busy massaging my lower back, and I insisted that Dwight call out the contraction time in five second intervals. The focus time for me was 15 seconds, because I told myself that was the contraction climax time and from then the pain would subside. I told myself I was strong enough to endure fifteen seconds of pain—15 seconds wasn't much time—and then I'd have about two pain-free minutes. Dwight's primary job was telling me the time. I'd grunt "time" when the contractions started. I knew Dwight was making up the time, but that somehow wasn't so critical as hearing the number 15.

After being freed from the monitoring device, the nurse encouraged me to take a shower. If I hadn't known I wanted to have an epidural, I probably would have wanted to deliver the baby in the shower. A chair was placed in the shower, and Dwight changed into the red bathing trunks I'd packed for him. I had two different positions—sitting hunched over or standing hunched over with my knee on the seat. As I had contractions, I told myself the water was washing away my stress and taking the pain down the drain. I tried to visualize my cervix opening.

I have no idea how long I was in the shower, but eventually we decided the doctor should check and see how I was progressing. I had made some progress, but not enough for the epidural; plus I was told several other women were in labor as well who also needed the anesthesiologist. Earlier, they had asked me to rate the pain from one to ten and I'd said eight. What a strange and annoying question to ask someone in labor! I wondered whether the anesthesiologist would have given me a higher priority if I had said ten.

A nurse brought in a rocking chair and encouraged me to try it out. It was a really comfortable chair with a footrest. When the contractions came, I'd push off the footrest and rock myself as I breathed deeply. For all the emphasis on breathing in the Lamaze classes, I don't know how you could go through labor without breathing like that—who could hold their breath through a contraction? When the contraction subsided, I went into a slumped, semi-sleep mode with my eyes feeling like they were weighed down by rocks.

When the doctor checked me again, I'd made progress and was lucky enough that the anesthesiologist was now available. I wondered if I was in a race with all these other women, and if so how I was doing. It took a while for the anesthesiologist to set up—it seemed like forever—though I'm sure it was only a matter of minutes.

The process of getting the epidural was rather straightforward and impersonal, and it took about 50 minutes for it to take effect. When it did, it was heavenly. I could see the contractions on the monitor, but not feel them. I was able to relax and even took a nap. Later, when the labor/delivery photos were developed, I saw that Dwight and Barbara had been playing around while I was sleeping, taking funny pictures of me. I'm glad they were in such high spirits so late at night.

After two hours, the doctors examined me and found I was effaced and almost completely dilated; but my water had not broken so she broke it for me with what looked like a crochet hook. Then I was told it was time to push. They helped me pull my knees to my chest and I held onto them with both hands. When they said "push," I'd take a deep breath and breathe down, imagining I was having a bowel movement. I wondered if all the constipation during pregnancy was preparation for this moment.

Since I couldn't feel a thing, they had to tell me when to start and when to stop pushing. They'd placed an internal monitor on the baby's head, and Dwight and Barbara could see my progress based on the movement of the monitor cord in and out of my body. When the baby's head was visible, Barbara moved the freestanding mirror so that I could see for myself. The doctor said the baby's head was big, and I should be glad I had the epidural. We'd brought Barbara's video camera intending to film immediately after the delivery, but Barbara suddenly decided to capture the moment right then. Somehow she was able to hold the camera and watch directly at the same time. The video she took is really wonderful, and I've enjoyed watching it. At home soon after the baby's birth, friends wanted to watch the video when they visited, and we were all crying at the end. I've been trying to pinpoint why we cry. Maybe it's simply the miracle and wonder of life—and not just this life, but our own as well. At that particular moment of birth, you can't help but think that this is something you went through once with your mother. It's a journey we've all taken.

At 7:04 a.m., the doctor told me not to push, but hum. It's funny that after all that pushing, my soft humming was what delivered Aaron into the world. I hope this means his introduction to the world was a gentle one, and his life will be a gentle, though of course not uneventful, one.

When he was lifted onto my stomach, I thought, "This is him—this is the moment we've been waiting for." Later, Dwight said that at this moment you realize that through the pregnancy you look at the labor as a termination point, but at the moment of birth you realize you've really been waiting for the beginning. (It sounded much more profound when he said it and we'd been up all night!)

Once your child is born, you feel every positive emotion at once— joy, love, relief, excitement, optimism, energy; I guess that's why in labor you feel every negative sensation—pain, fear, fatigue, anxiety. The duality counter-balances the focused moment of the miracle of birth. I think during labor I was in touch with the positive forces–the anticipation and excitement of knowing our introduction was imminent–and that's what pulled me through it all.

After Aaron was born, they placed him on my stomach. The doctor gave Dwight the largest scissors I'd ever seen and he cut the cord. I was so exhausted and I knew Dwight was too, so the scissors really scared me, and I was relieved when they were away from the baby.

One of the nurses took the baby to a side area, made sure he was okay, and then gave him a bath. Aaron was like a wet rag in the bath, slumped over and dazed, but he seemed to enjoy the experience of his first bath. With the epidural still in effect, the afterbirth seemed to just happen without me even being aware of it.

When it was all over, they brought Aaron to me, and I nursed him while lying on my side. It was very exciting to have him on my breast and to see him. I'd thought I'd recognize him immediately from telepathic messages in my dreams, but I didn't. His face was much rounder than I'd expected, and he had a lot of hair. I did recognize his nose right off, but his eyes and mouth were hard to place.

What helped me in terms of labor:
1. Dwight calling out contraction time in five second intervals—my focus was 15 seconds because I told myself 15 seconds was the climax time, and from there the pain would subside.
2. Hot shower— imagining water washing stress and pain down the drain.

3. Roller massage on my lower back—the sensation distracted my mind from some of the pain of the contractions.
4. Listening to music that I was very familiar with.
5. Sitting in the rocking chair.
6. Sugar-free lemon drops and lots of water.
7. Looking at photos of happy and relaxed times together, reminiscing about happy times, walking through memories.
8. Changing positions frequently and moving around.

    —*Proud mommy Beverly*

The Prolonged Labor

I have had two children, born 25 months apart. Both deliveries were vaginal. I characterize the birth of my first child as arduous and a bit of a nightmare. The birth of my second child was closer to the norm I hear described by other mothers.

My first delivery was after a prolonged labor. I was exhausted. I had been up for two nights in a row with labor that did not progress, but prevented me from getting any sleep. By the time I had dilated enough to push, I was wiped out from natural exhaustion and the oral sedatives that I had received earlier to help me sleep. My labor was weak, and I was put on a pitocin drip. A vacuum extractor was used to help deliver the baby.

I was very sore for days after the delivery. The difficult time I experienced during labor and immediately postpartum was amplified by my inability to breast-feed successfully. Despite lactation consultation and frequent pumping, my milk just never seemed to "come in." Due to inadequate weight gain by the baby, within a month's time I abandoned breast-feeding altogether.

By comparison, labor with my second child progressed more "normally," and he was born within eleven hours of the start of labor. An epidural was administered to help with pain relief. Similar to the first birth, the baby's head seemed lodged in the birth canal. This time, forceps were used to help delivery. I experienced the same breast-feeding issues as with the first baby and gave up on breast-feeding within a month.

Prior to the birth of our first child, my husband and I took the full battery of labor/delivery, breast feeding, and infant care courses available through our medical center. These courses were excellent, but did not mentally prepare me for coping with prolonged labor or the emotional roller coaster caused by breast feeding problems. I feel that my experiences in both of these arenas were far worse than the "average" of other mothers I have consulted.

Because of the exhaustion with my first delivery, my primary emotion was relief to have the baby born (at last!). In the case of the second, quicker delivery, I felt more like myself and was able to enjoy the newborn more. My most memorable moment of the birth process came with the delivery of my second baby. I recall the anesthesiologist speaking to me before administering the epidural. I'm sure they are required by regulations to ensure that patients understand the potential risks of the medication, but I was in no mood to listen to the details. I thought, "Yeah, yeah, yeah, just shut up and give me the !@#$% shot already!"

—*Proud mommy Susan*

Three Different Births

My name is Ann, and I have three beautiful children: Michael, Nicholas and Catrina. Michael is four, Nicholas is three and Catrina is two. I had a somewhat different birth experience with each of my children, but looking back on them now, I don't think I would have changed a thing.

With your first, you're not quite sure what to expect. My husband, Gaetano, and I went to all of the prenatal classes and hospital tours that you are expected to go to. It seems like I read every prenatal book on the shelves.

Michael was born ten days early. We were completely unprepared with not a single bag packed; in fact, I was supposed to be at work that day. Michael started his journey into the world at approximately 5 a.m. I got up to go to the bathroom and didn't quite make it. It was not a gush of water. So was it my waters breaking or was I incontinent? (By the way, bladder control is one of those little pregnancy "things" they don't always talk about, but I lost it towards the end of each pregnancy and for a few weeks after each vaginal delivery. My husband was buying diapers for the newborns and for me!) Soon after my waters broke, my contractions started. They were mild, but definitely present at first, and then began getting much stronger.

Being new at this, Gaetano and I weren't quite sure when to go to the hospital. So we packed our bags and rushed out the door. We arrived at the hospital at 7 a.m. After two hours of mild contractions, I thought for sure I would be at least six centimeters dilated. The nurse did my initial exam, and I was barely a meager three centimeters with a long way to go.

Once we were admitted to a room, Gaetano and I did a lot of walking. We walked the halls for hours. Walking, above all, helped me the most. The pain and the strength of the contractions steadily grew. The doctor pumped me full of pitocin because she "didn't want me to be in labor for a long time." I thank her for that! The staff asked a few times whether I wanted an epidural. I kept refusing, thinking I would ask for one after the next contraction. Well, for all three of my deliveries I kept saying that to myself, and I got to the point when it was time to push. Oh what a relief that was! After twelve hours of labor and fifteen minutes of pushing, we had our first of three beautiful babies.

Michael was born at 5:15 p.m. The doctor who was on the floor during the day and the nursing staff were fabulous. I think staffing dictates a lot about how your personal experience will be. Without the wonderful support I received from my husband, family, friends and hospital staff, my birth experiences wouldn't have been as wonderful as they were.

My experience with Nicholas' birth was much the same. I don't mean to disregard the middle child, but my waters broke, I had contractions immediately following and he was born about nine hours later. Nicholas was quite the surprise—he was born three weeks early. And to think we weren't prepared for Michael; we really were not prepared for Nicholas.

Catrina's birth day was a little bit different. By the time the third one comes around, we are pros at this, right? I woke up at around 8 a.m. Fathers' Day morning with contractions that were noticeable and regular. I sat on the sofa for awhile and decided that this was for real. I got Gaetano out of bed; we got the boys ready for a Fathers' Day celebration at their grandparents' house and a two-night sleepover. Then we were off. After we dropped the kids off, we went to Radio Shack and bought a battery for the camcorder, and then went to the deli to get Gaetano a sandwich for the long haul ahead. I'll never forget the reaction the deli cashier gave us when he asked what are plans were for this beautiful sunny day. Gaetano's response was, "We're walking down the block to the hospital to have a baby." The cashier's mouth almost hit the floor. I guess you don't hear that every day.

We arrived at the hospital at 1 p.m. This time, I really thought for sure I was at six centimeters. Nope, I was at two and a half. They weren't sure if they wanted to admit me. However, with a little begging, they were persuaded. I was told things were progressing so slowly because my waters hadn't broken. So they broke my waters. This, to me, was the worst part of all three of my birth experiences. They break your waters with this devise that looks like a crochet hook. I suppose this is easy and painless if they can do it on the first or second attempt, but that wasn't the case for me. My breathing exercises came in real handy as I was lying on the table staring at the ceiling for what seemed like hours. I'm sure it was only ten minutes. The staff was able to get the job done.

After my waters were broken, the contractions came fast and furious. The hours of bliss I enjoyed earlier were interrupted by hard labor. Catrina was born at 8:30 p.m. All of the staff knew we had two boys, and we were all hoping for a girl. Everyone cheered when a healthy little girl was born. It was a really neat experience.

All of my birth experiences were a little different, somewhat tedious, enlightening, but for the most part amazing! And I would do it again in a heartbeat (much to the dismay of my husband). We have so many wonderful things to look forward to, and I am forever grateful for what I have!

—*Proud mommy Ann*

THE BIRTH OF MY FIRST CHILD

My son, Larson, is my first child. He was born on April 12, 1997 when I was 35 years old. From the very beginning, my pregnancy went very well. I credit my active lifestyle and psychological readiness to be a mom with the relatively low level of physical discomfort that I experienced during my pregnancy. At the time I became pregnant, I had been running and weight lifting three to four days per week for most of my adult life and continued with my typical workouts until about the fifth month of pregnancy, at which point I stopped running and started swimming. I also knew that a high level of fitness would help me during labor, delivery and recovery, as well. The weightlessness and gracefulness I felt in the water was wonderful.

I had done lots of reading (*What to Expect When You're Expecting* and a few other books and videos), but took no special classes on labor and delivery. I was taking enough other classes at the time—trying to finish my master's thesis before my son was born. All the reading I had done had convinced me that I wanted to do three things during my delivery: be in water to relieve the pressure; be walking and active as long as possible; and give birth with the aid of gravity (squatting, not lying down). I also wanted to be in the hospital for as short a time as possible. (My husband, Steven, a kidney transplant recipient, had already spent too much stressful time in the hospital, and I felt it would be better for all of us to be at home.)

I also trusted that my body was ready for this kind of experience—it was designed for childbirth; I would know what to do when the time came, and I had a relatively high tolerance for pain. I would deal with the pain of childbirth without drugs.

Because of what they called "advanced maternal age," Steven and I chose to have amniocentesis. We hadn't originally planned to learn the gender of our baby, but we thought that if someone in a lab was painstakingly laying out the chromosomes and the information would be available, well then, we might as well find out. When we discovered that we had a boy, we named him Larson and from then on we spoke to him, sang to him, and called him by his name.

I had hoped that I could finish my master's thesis before Larson was born, and the deadline imposed by his due date proved to be perfect. I delivered my revised, signed thesis to the graduate department at San Jose State on a Thursday; rested and had a wonderful meal with good friends on Friday, had a good night's sleep; and began labor about 9 a.m. Saturday morning.

When labor began, I spent the first hours wondering if this was really it, and went car seat shopping—a minor detail that had been overlooked in my rush to get my thesis finished. By noon, I felt the pains coming regularly and called my doctor to ask when I should come in to the hospital. "Soon" was the reply. I then interrupted my husband, who was conducting a faculty meeting. We arrived at the hospital by 2 p.m.

I remember being surprised that labor hurt so much during a contraction and not at all in between. I remember being annoyed when they put an IV in my arm and the fetal heart monitor around my belly. So much for the purely natural childbirth I had imagined—which I now realize is practically impossible in a hospital setting. I remember being happier than I expected to just lay there on the bed moaning and breathing during the most difficult labor. Steven tells me that I gripped his hand so tightly that I almost bruised it. I also remember asking my nurse at around 6 p.m., when I was experiencing particularly strong back labor, "What about something for the pain?" Her response was perfect for me, "Honey, you don't need anything for the pain. You're going to have this baby in two hours!"

She proved to be right. When I was fully dilated and the doctor had arrived, everyone said "push," and I did—only three times. On the third push, Larson exploded into the doctor's arms. It was 8 p.m. I had torn a bit in that final push and was pretty weak because I had a low white cell count, but I did feel relieved to have what seemed to be the hard part over with. We ordered Japanese takeout, and I have never tasted such delicious Miso soup in all my life. We got to sleep and had a decent night's rest except for the middle of the night scare when the nurses took Larson supposedly to do some kind of test after we had specifically stated that he should be with one of us at all times. Steven was livid.

The most magical moment for our family came when the nurses put Larson on my chest. His eyes were closed, and when Steven said his name, Larson immediately opened his eyes and looked directly into his father's. We were convinced that he knew who we were and who he was.

I will do a few things differently if we decide to have another child. I will find a midwife and attempt to have the birth either at home or a birthing center with less intervention. I will have Larson and my mother and mother-in-law as involved as possible in the process. I'm lucky that I can consider these options because my first childbirth went so smoothly. And as before, I will continue to stay fit and active to ensure that my body will be prepared.

—*Proud mommy Mara*

Now It's My Turn

I paced the floors at 1 a.m., careful not to awaken my sleeping husband.... I knew it was true labor, so I had a bath and relaxed as best I could. I mentally rehearsed my birth plan before having breakfast and going to the hospital at 6:30 a.m.

Having worked as a midwife for many years, childbirth was already a special part of my life. I was always intrigued at the marvel of a new life arriving into our world.

As a young midwife, I met a lady who wore red socks during her labor. She was very calm, breathed easily through every contraction, said she didn't really feel any pain, then she pushed her baby out with what seemed just a little effort. I have never forgotten her. I wondered if my own birth experience could be like hers.

After a normal, uneventful pregnancy, my delivery time was near. I had spent some time on my birth plan and ensured my husband understood all my requests. His copy was placed with his wallet and the car keys, and the other was placed in my bag along with my lip salve, moisturizer, etc.

On arrival at the hospital, we were greeted by a few of my colleagues who refused to believe I was in labor because I was still smiling. I was, however, but the smiling soon ceased. I needed a pair of red socks and pain relief. After my epidural, I was actually feeling like conversing with my nurse and my husband, and enjoying myself. Many contractions later, a sudden decrease in the fetal heart caused a "flurry" of activity in the room, and I was quickly prepared for a cesarean section. Meconium-stained amniotic fluid was present. A return to normal of the fetal heart was a sweet sound to my ears; the cesarean section was put on hold and an amniotic infusion commenced (to dilute the thick particulate meconium to decrease the risk of aspiration into the baby's lungs). I continued to labor with an oxygen mask on my face.

After a 15 hour labor, I pushed out a baby girl. It was an experience that is life changing and amazing. It was uniquely mine, as it is for every woman.

One of the most interesting aspects of my labor was the realization that the mother is somewhat disengaged from reality and partners should be advocates during childbirth.

My labor plan never actually made it out to my bag; my lip salve and moisturizer did! I was not like the lady who wore the red socks, but I was the mother of a beautiful baby girl.

My second pregnancy resulted in a planned, elective cesarean section delivery … but that's another story.

—*Proud mommy Martina*

A TWIN BIRTH

Because I was having twins, I decided to be induced at 38 weeks and four days (the four days are important, as I am proud and grateful for every day I carried those rascals!). My OB/GYN told me that once I hit 38 weeks, I could be induced if I so desired. At my 37 week appointment, I told him to schedule the birth for the following week, as I could barely walk and getting out of bed was a lengthy and painful ordeal.

We arrived at the hospital at 7 a.m. I was so afraid they would send me home because they did not have room, but we got to stay. As my OB and I agreed, the induction would be initiated by the breaking of my water. We would give the babies time to see if they wanted out, and then, if I was not making progress, we would talk about pitocin. I was induced with Cervidil from my first pregnancy, and it gave me a very high fever; I did not want to do that again.

At about 10 a.m., an OB came in and broke my water. She then reached under the sheets to check my dilation and she told me that she felt a little hand! (William's hand!) So she pushed that hand back up so it would not get in his way. First she said I was already dilated to three, then she said, "No make that four…. Oh, I can stretch her to five." Oddly, none of this hurt at all.

Anyway, the painless contractions I had been having for weeks continued and got a little stronger. I was planning to have an epidural, so the labor nurse, Peg, kept coming in and asking if I wanted my epidural. But for reasons I can't explain and can only be grateful for, I was not in pain. Finally, when I reached seven-centimeter dilation, I began to feel some slight pain (nothing like the first time); Peg suggested I get the epidural before it really started hurting. That made sense to me, so I went for it.

After the epidural, things started going downhill. First my blood pressure dropped precipitously and alarms kept going off. Peg was trying to look calm, but she could not keep her eyes off the blood pressure monitor. The anesthesiologist came in and gave me a shot of "epi," and my pressure rose some, but not as much as they would have liked. Finally they rolled me onto my right side and my pressure went back to normal. Unfortunately, because I was on one side, the epidural medication only went to one side of my body, so I could feel my now painful contractions on my left side.

The anesthesiologist gave me more medication, and my legs turned to lead. Shortly after that, my new labor nurse told me that I was ready to push. I was not ready for anything. My legs felt like lead, and I had no sensation from the waist down. I tried to push a few times, and it was so frustrating. I knew my pushing was totally ineffective. Suddenly, I began to fear that I would have to have a C-section. I started to cry. Mark reassured me that I had only just started and would get the hang of it. I did, but it took about 45 minutes before I gave a decent push.

After about 30 minutes of effective pushing, my OB came in and told me to stop pushing (Ha!). Mark put on his blue scrubs, and we went off to the operating room. Twins are delivered in the OR no matter what because they are considered high risk and the team wants to be ready in case anything goes wrong. Unlike when V was born, there was a cold, bright room with about six other people in it. I had to scoot over onto an operating table, where I was flat on my back until I finally asked someone if I could be tilted up a little. Once everyone was assembled and set up, they allowed me to resume pushing. That was about 20 minutes.

A few contractions later, William emerged. He was mad! My OB, always the comedian, said, "Hey, this one is a girl." I knew he was joking, but the nurses were giving him a quizzical look. They held Will up to show me, and then took him to a warming table to be checked by a neonatologist. She said he was fine, and they swaddled him. He stopped crying immediately. I was crying again, but this time I was happy.

As soon as Will came out, another OB began pushing down on the top of my uterus to guide Henry down and keep him from exploring his new, larger living space. I watched Will on the warming table ten feet away, and everyone else watched me. They were waiting for the contractions to resume. After about eight minutes, I felt a contraction, and I decided that it was time for Henry to come out. I pushed with every ounce of strength I had left and out he came. He was quiet for a minute, and then let everyone know how he felt about what had just happened. They checked my Henry out and he was fine, too. I have never been so relieved in my whole life. I felt so lucky, so blessed. And so hungry!

After Henry was swaddled, they brought both babies to me for a minute, and then Mark and the babies went to the nursery.

Prior to the boys' birth, we took a class about parenting twins offered by my hospital. After their birth, I met several times with Sarah, a lactation consultant who specializes in twins.

I think the most memorable moment came about 90 minutes after the boys were born. Unlike V's birth (my daughter), I did not get to hold the boys right when they were born. I looked at them for about 30 seconds, and then they were off to the nursery. I was wheeled back to my room and spent about 20 minutes alone while all the grandparents and V looked at the newest family members getting baths, etc. Finally, after more than an hour, Mark brought the boys in and handed them to me. It was wonderful. I finally got to see the little people I had worried so much over. I finally got to hold them after working so hard to bring them safely into the world. I don't have the words to describe how I felt, but of course I was crying. I will never forget that moment. V climbed up onto my bed and I had the three people who mattered most in the world on my lap. I was supremely happy.

If I ever have another baby (and I won't!), I think I would try it without the epidural. It was a great thing for V's birth, but with the boys, it just complicated everything. The pain I was in with V was excruciating, but I think I could have stood it if my labor had been shorter. Eventually, the pain just wore me down. Second labors are shorter.... I think I could have done it.

—*Proud mommy Nicole*

The Birth of a Daughter

Our daughter was born one week early. I saw my obstetrician on a Friday. On Saturday morning, I realized that my water broke. We went to the hospital, but I was sent home because I was not experiencing contractions close together. Early Sunday morning, we went back to the hospital because I was experiencing uncomfortable back labor. Although my contractions were still far apart, I was admitted to the hospital because I started throwing up. This continued throughout the day and evening. Although I was advised that the epidural would slow down my labor, I decided to go ahead with it. Given my fear of having a needle put in my back, the anesthesiologist was very sensitive and hid all the equipment from me during the procedure. (The next day, he came to visit me to make sure I had no ill effects from the epidural.) After several hours of pushing (lying down on my back), the doctor thought it was best to do a cesarean. I was prepped, but before doing my cutting, the doctor determine I had dilated enough, and that the baby's head was emerging naturally. After several hours of pushing, I was ready to have the cesarean procedure, but was glad when it turned out I didn't need it. Because we didn't know if we were having a boy or a girl, the mystery kept me going throughout the very long day. Considering the enormity of the situation, I was very calm. It was hard to sleep even with the pain medication, probably because I was so excited that our baby was finally being born. I thought the lead nurse was very sensitive and supportive, as was the anesthesiologist. My obstetrician was very confident and calming, even though she ended up delivering six babies over the course of a few hours that evening. I felt very comfortable with these people.

Before getting the epidural, I stood in the shower with the water running on my back to relieve the pain of the back labor. Once I got the epidural, however, I wasn't very mobile and just lay in the bed. Although I had decided to have an obstetrician deliver our baby, I could have had a midwife. University of California San Francisco (UCSF) is pretty supportive in this regard. The birthing rooms are very large. During the hours I pushed, the bed was tilted up to assist me, but not to the point that I was vertical with the floor.

We took classes in parenting, labor prep and infant nutrition. There were no classes offered to us after delivery, but I took a new mother's class at the Jewish Community Center.

We played music. I knew that I would be in a room with a lovely view of San Francisco, which also helped make the labor process more relaxing.

The most memorable moment of the whole birth experience was finding out that we had a healthy baby girl. If I were to have another baby, I would hold out longer before getting an epidural.
— Proud mommy Kim

Our Daughter's Birth

The year before I gave birth to Katy Rae, I had the educational experience of participating in the delivery of my good friend's baby. I took a birth/breathing class with her and her husband in preparation for the birth of their first child. When it came time to prepare for the delivery of my own child, I felt like I already knew the basics and that the rest was so individual that I would learn what I needed from the nurses.

As a result, David, my husband, and I did not take a prenatal class. In retrospect, I think a prenatal class would have been very helpful for my husband, who wasn't quite sure what to expect during Katy Rae's delivery. We did pre-register with the birth hospital and did a walk-through of the hospital, a process that I highly recommend for any parents-to-be.

For seven years before getting pregnant, I was living in Berkeley, and my OB/GYN was affiliated with a hospital in Oakland, California. While I had moved to San Francisco and was living in the city during my pregnancy, I didn't want to change doctors. Consequently, I spent the entire pregnancy wondering whether I would go into labor at 3 p.m. on a Friday during the height of rush hour and deliver Katy Rae on the Bay Bridge!

The week before Katy Rae was born, I had gone on maternity leave, prepared her bedroom, and selected a pediatrician. I was, therefore, looking forward to a week relaxing around the house before going into delivery. However, I went into labor 10 days earlier than my due date. On a beautiful weekend day, I was comfortably ensconced at home but for having the "false" contractions. I had been experiencing "false" contractions since my seventh month, so it was no surprise that I had been having them that day as well.

Sometime in the mid-afternoon, I discovered that I was bleeding very slightly. I immediately reviewed all of the labor/delivery books that I had accumulated. From what I could tell, the slight bleeding was not something to worry about, which was in line with my nature, as I'm not one to panic. At the time, David was out riding his bike, and by the time he came home I was bleeding like a light period. When I mentioned this to David, he said to call the doctor. It was around 6 p.m.

When the doctor returned my page, he told me very calmly, "Well, that sounds like something we should take a look at. What time would you like to meet at the hospital?"

We met our doctor at Alta Bates at around 8 p.m. I was certain the doctor would laugh at me because when we arrived I had not brought any clothes for Katy Rae or me, since I thought I would not be delivering Katy Rae for several more days. I also had not, at this point, really formulated a "birth plan" per se, so I had no idea what it would be like to be "the patient." I did, however, plan to walk around as much as possible during my eventual labor and try to deliver in an upright position.

The doctor did an ultrasound to find out why I was bleeding and admitted me for observation. As it turned out, I was WRONG, as I was in a very mild labor, which could have lasted for days or simply petered out. I ended up spending a very sleepless night in the hospital.

When the doctor came in the next morning, my labor had stopped, but I was still bleeding. The doctor then decided to induce my labor. Initially, the doctor broke my water. We waited one hour or so to see if that would jumpstart the process—it did not. Next, we graduated to pitocin. The doctor said the pitocin would take some time to work, so in the interim, he wanted to give me another medication to help me sleep.

Shortly thereafter, a nurse came in and started an IV. At first, I did not know what was in the IV; but when I started to become nauseated, I asked the nurse, who informed me the medication was morphine. I finally did get to sleep and actually slept for three to four hours. When I woke up, I felt "spaced out" and had a pounding headache. I was also quite nauseated from the morphine. I eventually got up to go to the restroom and unceremoniously vomited.

Anyway, the pitocin did its job quite rapidly, and I was in hard labor within five hours. I kept telling David I was in incredible pain, and I could hardly talk in the ten-second intervals between contractions. At some point, I screamed at my sister to get the nurse for me to do SOMETHING to relieve the incredible pain that was racking my entire body. I was then at seven+ centimeters, so the anesthesiologist arrived and administered an epidural. Unfortunately, for some reason, the epidural only worked on one side of my body.

Up to now, I had been in the hospital for 24 hours, and David had not left my side the entire time. The pained look on David's face made me wonder whether it was more excruciating to watch the delivery or to be the one giving birth! By 8 p.m., I was ten-centimeters dilated, but

I did not have the energy to keep pushing during contractions. The doctor was now back in the room and asked me to start pushing with each contraction. The nurses were counting out my breathing, and I was refocused on pushing. After what felt like five minutes, I looked at the clock and two hours had actually gone by! Time flies when you're having a "good" time?!

I looked around the room and realized that I had a huge audience of medical personnel. Starting with my doctor, his assistant and my nurse, there were now at least four more medical assistants witnessing the birth. When I asked if my baby was progressing toward my cervix, the doctor was nonresponsive and simply asked if I would like some "help" in expediting the delivery. My doctor proceeded to inform me that forceps would not work, but he could try to "suction" my baby out.

At this point, I started to panic a little. The suction cup popped off the baby's head the first time; the second time, I kid you not, the doctor put one foot on my bed for extra leverage. When he finally got the head out, I was looking at a beautiful head, totally blue. I was sure she was dead; David looked pretty concerned also. The doctor twisted her all the way around twice before getting her shoulder to drop enough to get her out; then she got stuck trying to get her tummy out. Finally, she was out, and everyone was so excited I had to ask if it was a boy or girl. The pediatrician took her immediately to make sure that she wasn't too traumatized.

After having the most incredible, healthy pregnancy, I really had expected a much easier birth. The whole experience made me realize that you never really know what will happen, even if you have been through it before. Each experience is unique.

My most memorable experience was definitely seeing her beautiful face the first time. I would go through that 24 hours of my life a thousand more times if I had to.

I was recently talking to my friend who is 34 weeks pregnant. We were talking about birth plans. I was telling her my only advice is to ask questions *before* things start happening and to know all the options—good and bad.

If we were to have another baby, I would have the epidural, but resist other drugs, such as morphine, if possible. I would also seriously look into a doula in order to be better informed about my choices and to have someone constantly present to advocate for me throughout my labor. (I was in labor at a very busy time and sometimes had a difficult time getting the attention of the nurses.)

—*Proud parents Sheri and David*

My Two Deliveries

Even before I had my two children, I was never very interested in hearing other women talk about their labor and delivery experiences. Maybe it's because, in my family, C-sections, not vaginal deliveries, were considered "natural." My mother had three C-sections and her sister had four. My brothers and I were all born at 8:30 a.m. on Monday mornings. My mother claims she was told that her hips were too narrow to attempt a natural delivery, but I've always suspected her male OB just didn't work weekends.

When I became pregnant with my daughter at age 36, my husband and I took the suggested course on natural childbirth, and at the time I remember thinking, "Okay, I can do this." At 30 weeks, my OB determined that our daughter was in a breech position. At 32 weeks, they attempted to turn her manually. That was the only time I experienced pain during that entire pregnancy and delivery. Fortunately, they made a halfhearted attempt, but it was still excruciating. There was a British nurse assisting that day and when the OB left the room, she turned to us and said, "My daughter was breech too, and I had a C-section. They don't do enough breech deliveries in this country to do it vaginally." We'd already been leaning toward having the C-section, and, at that point, we made the decision to leave natural childbirth behind permanently.

The scheduled C-section was done at 35 weeks, and it was a completely enjoyable experience. I walked to the operating room where they did the spinal. There was no pain at all. Elinor came out with a tiny cry and was instantly alert. She scored 9.9 on the Apgar scale. The anesthesiologist said it was, "the calmest birth I've ever attended." We had a doula in the operating room with us who kept me company after Elinor was delivered. My husband accompanied baby Elinor to the nursery.

There was one complication that surfaced about a week later. Apparently, I'd had an undiagnosed urinary tract infection when they did the surgery. The catheter pushed bacteria into the uterus to the kidneys, and I ended up with an infection. Ironically, I didn't pay attention to the wracking chills I was experiencing initially because a friend who had had her three children naturally had told me to expect them. In my case, they were signs of serious infection. It took three days of IV antibiotics to clear it up. Each day, I'd step carefully down the stairs with the doula and baby in tow. The infection threw my nursing off for a week or so, but after that everything was fine.

With my second pregnancy, I chose a scheduled C-section from the beginning. I'd had no adverse effects at all, and the first one had gone so well that I definitely wanted another. In fact, the prospect of natural childbirth actually gave me pause when we were deciding whether or not to have a second child. Just before we were set to start trying, my OB informed me that a recent study done at UCSF showed that vaginal birth for older mothers was often not advised. I said, "If you'll agree to do another section, I'll sign up for a second baby." She said, "I think we can arrange that." The second surgery went just as smoothly as the first. The surgery team stressed over and over that due to scar tissue and aging, the second surgery would take longer and could be more complicated. They were so emphatic about this that I was a little frightened going into the OR the second time. But there was no trouble at all. Both babies were born at 1:29 p.m. with surgery starting at 1 p.m. Matthew was born just as alert as Ellie and also scored 9.9 on the Apgar scale. And recovery the second time was uncomplicated. I spent a week in bed just as a precaution, but I had no pain at all.

I don't understand the politicizing of childbirth. Today when mothers sit and trade war stories about their birth experiences, I keep quiet. At least in [the San Francisco Bay Area], telling people you had two lovely, planned C-sections isn't wise. Women are militant about natural delivery, but to me it's all the same in the end. It's like focusing on the wedding instead of the marriage. In the end, it's the parenting that comes after the birth that really counts.

—*Proud mommy Sarah*

THE BIRTH OF A SON

I was in labor for 49 hours. We first went to the hospital at 3 a.m. I was having strong contractions that took me to the ground approximately five to ten minutes apart. We were told by one of the MDs on call that I was only one centimeter dilated. Prodromal labor is the term they use. I went home at 7:30 a.m. not to return until 9 p.m. It was a long day. I must admit that I sipped a little red wine at home to try to relax.

The midwife was very compassionate and gave me a shot of morphine (15m). I slept through the night, with another shot along the way to help me sleep.

When I woke up in the morning, I was only four cm dilated. The MD who examined me convinced me to be started on a pitocin drip. So the labor became more intense and my dilation was not quick. At around 2 p.m., I was exhausted. I was given 50 milligrams of fentanyl every hour. It was like giving me a shot of water. I had an epidural. Dead legs they call it. Now, all the monitors were on and flushing/beeping. The nurses were great. They, of course, were my advocates along the way.

The MD, at some point, offered me a cesarean. We were about 40 hours into this process; she was worried. I told her that if mom and baby were not in danger—NO WAY!

Around 8 p.m., I was dilated to ten cm. I held a towel around a bar that my feet rested on and pushed for the next two hours. The epidural was slowly wearing off. My legs grabbed the bar stronger with every push. I could feel my body more and more. The anesthesia doctor came in to give me more epidural medicine, but I said, "No thank you."

Around 10:30 p.m., Spencer was born—naturally. The medicine was not working anymore. In the end, I felt content.

I did not take any classes prior to delivery. We played music and lit candles at home for relaxation.

The most memorable moment was when they told me that I could start pushing. I don't know that I would do anything differently. I think the difference would unfold on its own.

—*Proud mommy Laurie*

A FATHER'S DELIVERY

When Carol was about 32 weeks along, she had some false contractions for which we spent an evening at the hospital with her hooked up to a monitor. The nurse was a veteran labor and delivery nurse named Pat. We liked her a lot. Over the course of the evening, Pat told us that her idea of the perfect hospital would be one with all nurses, no doctors. The doctors could be hired when it was really necessary, she explained. But mostly the nurses knew all they needed to know.

On a Sunday morning two weeks later, after a delicious breakfast of french toast, Carol left the table, went into the bathroom and said very clearly and calmly, "Oh, s***."

"Oh, s*** what, honey?" I asked.

"Oh s*** my water just broke," she said.

As this was only 34 weeks into the pregnancy, we were not packed for travel, and we had only taken three of the six birthing classes. We had no crib, no diapers, no baby supplies at all. But it was time to go. We called the hospital and they said to come right in, not only because her water had broken, but also because Carol had already had some difficulties with the pregnancy and had been on bed rest for a while. She cleaned up while I paced nervously and tried to pack for an indeterminate stay at the birth unit.

We arrived at the hospital around noon, as I recall. They did not seem too anxious to get us into a room, as Carol could not yet feel any contractions and the staff were quite busy. So we sat in the waiting room, walked the halls and tried to remain calm for a while. After about an hour, we were shown to our room. We told the nurse that we would like to have Pat for a nurse, and she said, "Oh good. Pat is coming on duty in just a little while." By the time she arrived, Carol was in the bed and hooked up to a couple of monitors. One was showing the contractions every few minutes.

"Can you feel that?" she asked Carol.

"Not yet."

By this time Sarah, Carol's best friend, had arrived. Pat took up a position near the door to ward off inquiring doctors.

"We're all set in here," Pat would say. "Everything is fine."

She explained to us that Carol belonged to them now, no matter what happened. Once the water breaks, the baby can theoretically stay in for a while; this is, however, extremely dangerous for all concerned, so Carol would have to lie on her back in the hospital for the duration, which could be weeks.

It was about 2:30 p.m. when Carol began to feel the contractions in a big way. Our birth class instructor, Maggie Greenwood, had told us in the first class that, in her opinion, special breathing techniques were overrated.

"Just try to relax your body as much as possible, and you will know how to breathe," she had said. Carol fell right into it. Also, I seem to remember that it was partly because of Maggie's influence that we had decided not to make a birth plan. We had decided that, while we wanted a natural birth, what we wanted most was a healthy baby.

In any event, because of Carol's superb physical condition and high tolerance for pain, she felt able to deal with the first strong pains without any drugs. I was the one who needed drugs. I was not prepared for how helpless and distressed I felt when Carol would have a contraction. It was very upsetting to see her in pain.

Sarah and I helped Carol maneuver from the bed to the shower and back. We kept the ice cup full. Pat came and went often, mostly to reassure me, I felt, that the various blips and bleeps on the monitors were nothing to worry about. I kept panicking when the heart monitor showed the baby's heart slowing down.

I was so uncomfortable I kept thinking of things back home that I thought we needed. But Sarah and Carol would not let me leave. I just wanted to get away from the distress. Carol, however, never seemed distressed. Waves of pain would hit her, but she found ways to ride them out.

At one point, the phone rang and I answered it. It was Carol's brother calling from Florida. He had heard that we had left for the hospital, and he thought he would call to see if there was any news yet. All the women in the room stared icily at me while I stammered something or other, then hung up.

Now I cannot remember the stages of the birth process, but Carol progressed through them all as in the textbook. Around 5 p.m. or so, she found a way to make a low moaning sound during the contractions. At this point, she was mostly kneeling on the bed with Sarah and me for support. When the contraction would hit, she would start this long, low-pitched "OOOOOOOOOOOOO" sound with each breath. It seemed to be soothing to her. I loved hearing this sound because I knew I would never hear it again.

As it became clear that she was moving toward having the baby soon, doctors began showing up. Because it was a premature birth, there was the resident physician, and then there was the head of the department, the premature pediatric team, and a few others near the end. Pat called the shots until just before the birth. She kept everyone out of the way so Carol could be free to have the baby her own way. Sometime after 5:30 p.m., perhaps 5:45, Carol began to push. She only pushed about four or five times when Pat said, "All right, there it is. Want to see it?" And she held a mirror so Carl could see the top of the baby's head. At that point, the crowd of doctors—I think there were five in all—took over the baby receiving duties. But Pat stayed near the center of the action and held Carol's hand.

Carol pushed again and out came the head. Rest. Pushed again, and out came an arm. Rest. Pushed again, and out flew a baby boy, all reddish gray. A nurse handed me some scissors and held up a clamped off section of the umbilical cord to cut. I cut.

From my point of view, the moment when the baby was born was not the most beautiful moment of my life or anything ecstatic. I was out of my head with fear and anxiety at seeing my wife in so much pain. This baby was what had been causing all the pain. I did not care so much about it at that moment, only about Carol and all she was going through.

Because the baby was premature, the doctors had to execute an elaborate checklist. The most amusing was "Bonding," where they laid the baby on Carol's chest for one minute, I think. Check. Bonded. Then they took him away to the nursery, where they could watch him every moment for 24 hours.

When I looked at the clock, it was 6:30 p.m., four hours from the time Carol felt the first contractions. The baby weighed five and a quarter pounds. We did not give him a name for a week or so. Finally, we named him Jules, after Carol's grandmother Julia.

The first three weeks of Jules' life were terrible because he had a birth defect no one detected. He had a spot where his intestines grew together, a "duodenal stenosis." So he could not absorb food. Finally, after great tribulation, they figured out the problem and called in a renowned surgeon to operate on Jules, curing his stenosis and his hernias. From then on he was serious about eating and growing, and is now one of the largest, healthiest boys in his class.

—*Proud daddy Joe*

An Enjoyable Birth

The birthing experience was a very comfortable and enjoyable one for us. The hospital provided us with a very agreeable suite with a private bathroom. By the time I was admitted into the hospital, I was in quite considerable pain and was waiting for my epidural to arrive. The doctors and nurses were very available and supportive. After receiving the epidural, I calmed down well and remember being able to participate and enjoy the whole experience of giving birth to our daughter. When the time came to actually deliver Karishma, my OB/GYN came well prepared. She was joking, laughing, supporting and reassuring us all at the same time. She would give explicit instructions and we would follow. With that came Karishma, who arrived well and safely. It was indeed a beautiful feeling to hold your baby at last after all the waiting and working. I don't remember feeling nervous or scared, only that all would be well soon.

We had taken childbirth and child care classes during the time of our older daughter, Mehek, so we did not feel the need to retake the classes. We were invited to join a parents group after Karishma was born, but chose against it as we had enough support and help from family members.

We did not light candles as such but we did keep a profound "Food Log" for her. We recorded everything we ate on a daily basis and placed it under the various food categories. It was a very rewarding and fun experience, and ensured the that we ate the highest quality food. I also managed to drink at least two liters of water daily more often than not.

The most memorable moment for me was right after Karishma's arrival. It was when all the family had left for home and I was alone with my baby for the very first time. I will never forget the overwhelming love I felt for her. I stared at her for a long time, admiring the miracle God had given to us and seeing how perfect she was in every sense. It was love at its best. I thought I would burst with happiness and fulfillment. She was just so beautiful. The only other time I have felt this powerful force of Nature - Love was when I held Mehek under the same circumstances two years ago.

I don't think I would do anything differently for my daughters, as I felt it was the best I'd given of myself to them during and after the pregnancy.

Thank you for letting me share my experience with you.

—*Proud mommy Mona*

Birth with a Doula

There was no doubt in my mind that I would have a doula at the birth of my second child. My husband had doubts. Or rather, he thought it was a "waste of time." But he kept these thoughts to himself until nearly eight months after the birth of our second daughter, Jessica. He knew that I was stubborn—there would be a doula at the birth, end of discussion.

I had a right to be stubborn (or so I thought). My first birthing experience ended in a cesarean 44 hours after my water broke and 12 hours after my body didn't respond to pitocin. Throughout those 44 hours, I felt disconnected—I remember thinking if only my brain and body could be connected, everything would be okay. Four years later, when I became pregnant again, I still felt that way: if only my brain and body had been connected, I wouldn't have had a cesarean.

We found a list of doulas in our area by entering our zip code into the Doulas of North America (DONA) website. From the list of over 30 names, I contacted five via e-mail and we interviewed three. I selected one (I gave my husband veto power!) who I felt was most like me.

What I liked best about the doula we selected was that she viewed this experience as a team experience. She immediately had several ideas to help us when she found out that we wanted to include our four-year-old daughter in the birthing experience.

We hired her when I was about three months along and we met with her at our house for an hour once a month. During the first few meetings, we got to know each other and she asked us questions pertaining to our birth plan. In the last three or four meetings, my husband (and sometimes our daughter) and I would do relaxation techniques that she would guide us through. And when we went on the hospital tour, she went with us as well.

I liked the fact that we really got to know her, and I felt comfortable within a couple meetings that she would be able to be a good birthing advocate—which is really how I view a doula, someone to support you and to promote your plan. The best way I could explain it to my friends was this: "She's the brains and I'll do the physical work."

After working with a doula, I revised the longing that I had to have my brain and body connected during my first birth—I believe now that the birthing experience is a very physical task and my brain actually might have been too much in the way. Your brain needs to be connected but focused on only one thing—birthing (or, in some instances, blocking out the pain!). The doula will do everything else.

Our doula was amazing. She was with us, by our side, for over 40 hours! I had mostly back labor and it helped for my husband or her to press on the lower part of my back. This went on for about 12 hours, so, like me, they were both exhausted after the birth. On the way home from the hospital, my husband would comment on how it was a good thing there was someone else to help with the physical aspects of being the birthing coach.

Because of our meetings during the pregnancy, I was able to relax knowing that she would be our advocate for our birth plan. I could just focus on managing the pain and birthing our daughter.

It was an incredible experience. I was able to meet all my birthing goals. My husband recently told me, "I was just going along [with having a doula] because you wanted it; I thought it was a waste of time, but it turned out pretty good. It was especially good to have someone there who knew what they were doing and who wasn't emotionally attached." I couldn't agree more. When I reflect on that experience, I am in awe of our doula's talents and how she put them to use for us.

—*Proud mommy Timi*

HOME BIRTH

I delivered my first baby in a hospital. Thanks to a lot of mental preparation, prenatal yoga, the support of my husband and a wonderful doula, I was able to labor and deliver drug free, something I wanted both for the baby's sake and for my own. I wanted to trust my body and experience the whole process of birth. While I was happy that I was able to birth naturally, my experience at the hospital was still very medical, impersonal, and guided by the protocols and routines of the hospital (being strapped to the fetal monitor, pushing in a semi-reclining position, etc.). The birth of my son seemed to take place according to their rules and on their timetable, not my own. In this sense, it wasn't very "natural" at all.

When I became pregnant with my second child, I decided to look into birthing at home attended by midwives. With home birth, I knew that I could have a softer, more peaceful environment in which to labor and welcome the baby to the world. While I knew that I couldn't control or pre-plan everything about the process (since each birth is so unique), I wanted to be surrounded by familiar faces rather than a rotating cycle of strangers. I found two great midwives, Chloe Ohme and Jen Bauman, who work as a team. From the very beginning, I noticed the difference between the midwife model of care and the traditional medical model. I felt like an active partner in the process, rather than a patient who had all my decisions made for me by a doctor. My appointments with Chloe and Jen were not the five-minute, assembly-line appointments I had had with my OB; we often met for an hour or more (at my house!), and our conversations were wide-ranging. We discussed everything from nutrition during pregnancy to how to manage the birthing process and what to do with my toddler. We talked about how memories I had about the last birth might affect the upcoming one. My husband was encouraged to come to the appointments.

I went into labor on a Monday afternoon. It was great to be able to have freedom of movement in familiar surroundings and all of the comforts of home. My husband timed the contractions and I was in constant contact with my midwives, who were ready to come over once the contractions were closer together. Throughout the afternoon, I did a lot of visualizations during the contractions. I used my yoga breathing and moaned "OM" as I imagined the cervix opening wide. I pictured the baby making his journey. I tried to concentrate on the wavelike motions of the contractions and take advantage of the breaks between them.

Around 8:30 p.m., we called Chloe and Jen. When they arrived, I was almost ready to start pushing, but even though things were getting intense for me, they exuded a calm, businesslike air as they made all of their preparations. I was amazed at how unobtrusive they were. They really let me stay in my moment and not get distracted. I was ready to start pushing around 10:30 p.m., and the midwives suggested that I get into the birthing tub. (We rented one from a woman who comes and sets it up in your home. We had it installed in our bedroom.) Being in the water was great. It definitely helped soften the tremendous thrust of gravity as the baby was moving down through the birth canal.

Our second baby boy was born shortly before midnight. Chloe pulled him out of the water and set him on my chest. We were both warm and wet and relaxed as we looked into each other's eyes for the first time. Then—and this is one of the great things about home birth—we all made our way to our own bed while the midwives checked the baby and me and cleaned up. When Chloe and Jen left several hours later, we were still on a high from witnessing our little miracle come into the world. We ate leftover pizza and peanut butter toast and made some phone calls to the grandparents. When we did finally rest, we were a family together in our own quiet house.

The excellent midwife care continued in the postpartum weeks. My midwives came to check on the baby and me three times in the first week, and then again at the third week and finally at week six.

Home birth is obviously not for everyone. I had a healthy, risk-free pregnancy. Chloe and Jen are trained to be on the lookout for potential risks that are beyond their scope, at which point they would have suggested I see the doctor. But for me, home birth was a great way to be an active participant in the most profound physical experience a woman can have. Being able to endure the hard work of labor without drugs or interventions has given me the confidence that I can withstand the toughest challenges. It has given me a source of strength that I routinely need to tap into as a mother of two beautiful boys.

—*Proud mommy Brigitte*

A FATHER'S PRIDE

I can remember it so vividly. The top of my daughter's head, Cliodhna, protruding slightly as my wife, Irene, red faced and exhaling controllably, clenched the white sheets of the bed. I was not merely a bystander, I was a participant as the nurse guided me through the process, all the while working closely with the doctor. It was as if we were in a bubble; the room was quiet other than the blinking, colorful lights of the machines evaporating in the dim of the room. I remember thinking how professional the two medical personnel were as I stood there holding my wife's hand and comforting her. As if synchronized, the nurse and the doctor moved fluidly as we all watched Cliodhna's face emerge. Irene's concentration did not waver even in the pain and discomfort she felt. The glow on her face showed determination as she continued to breathe like a machine. It seemed so agonizingly slow (even for me who had both legs planted firmly on the floor) when Cliodhna's entrance into the world seemed to slow down as her right shoulder did not want to come free.

More direction from the medical staff, encouraging Irene to continue to breathe and for Dad to help comfort her. Then, all of the sudden, Cliodhna emerged, shiny, arms flaying and gasping for breath as the doctor gave me the honor of cutting the umbilical cord. As they quickly swaddled our daughter, I remember thinking how strange it was that I had little apprehension, as if the birth was a stage play rehearsed to perfection—the medical staff never seemed to break a sweat.

I also clearly remember wondering why on earth a woman would accept this ordeal—the constant changes in the body and the twisting and contorting for nine months. But Irene's face divulged the answer as I stared at her, snuggling with the tightly swaddled Cliodhna and peppering her with small kisses. Irene's face was exhausted (whose face wouldn't be?), shiny pink from all the capillaries bursting with blood.

It was Irene's expression. Was it joy that the physical labor was over? Was it relief that the labor turned out well? I stood there and gaped at my family, feet stuck in concrete as the other medical staff came in on cue. It finally dawned on me. It was exuberant pride. Irene gave birth to a child. A beautiful baby girl, slightly confused at her new surroundings, who automatically clung to her mother as her face snuggled into the nook of Irene's shoulder. As if choreographed, the bond was set as Cliodhna blinked at her mother. Irene fully comprehended this feeling, as if they were siamese twins. No words were spoken, they were not needed. Irene's facial expression said it all.

Would I want to go through the physical labor of having a baby? Absolutely not, but it has always been noted that women are tougher than men are. But if I can again share and participate in the moment of seeing my child emerge into the world, I will be there in a flash with bells and whistles.

—*Proud daddy Timothy*

BIRTH WITH A MIDWIFE

For me, working with a Certified Nurse Midwife and a Lay Midwife were two of the most empowering relationships that I have had, and I am grateful for the guidance and expertise that they both brought me, my husband and my family during the birth of my two children.

When I became pregnant with my first child, I was in San Francisco and far away from my Maine family and friends. I talked to several doctors, visited all the labor and delivery units in local hospitals and discovered that there were no birth centers in San Francisco where a woman and her family could labor and deliver with the least amount of intervention from medical technology. This was a key point for me, as I felt like I appreciated all that the medical community could offer, but that I did not want the delivery of my child to be a medical procedure. Two new friends had recently had babies, and they told me about their plans for home births with their midwives, which was an entirely new concept for me. As I started talking with various midwives, my husband and I came to realize that a home birth would be the best way for us to bring our new baby into the world.

After meeting with several midwives with very different backgrounds and styles, my husband and I decided that choosing a Certified Nurse Midwife, Kathryn Newburn, to assist us in a home birth would work best for us. Kathryn's midwifery training and experience, coupled with her nursing background and certifications, helped us feel like we were bringing together the best of both worlds—medical expertise combined with a midwife's holistic approach. The personal care and attention that I got from working with her was a great source of strength, knowledge and deeper appreciation for the process of growing a healthy baby. When I went into labor at home, having Kathryn and her assistants with my husband and me truly helped us feel in control and prepared to have a healthy and safe delivery. After 46 hours of labor, it was she who helped me make the decision to transport to a hospital and ultimately to have a C-section birth. Having a midwife working with me before, during and after the birth of my son was a very empowering and joyful experience. Even though I had a C-section in the end, I felt that my wishes and needs were heard and addressed at every step of the way, which was the only way for me to be able to move through this huge transition in my life successfully.

When I became pregnant with my second child there was no doubt in my mind that I wanted to work with a midwife and try to do a home birth again. I had some trepidation as to whether this was the safest choice for me and the baby, so I talked again with several doctors, certified nurse midwives and lay midwives—women and men who delivered babies exclusively in hospitals and others who delivered babies exclusively at home. I was concerned about the fact that I was 38 years old and had a previous C-section. Everyone agreed that I was not at risk, and that there was no reason why I would not be able to have a perfectly normal delivery either at home or in the hospital. So I chose a midwife, Maria Iorillo, to work with me to prepare for and deliver my baby at home. Again, working with an experienced and grounded midwife like Maria was so empowering, strengthening, and, in many ways, healing for me. As it turned out, my second baby was breech, and despite every effort imaginable to turn her around she remained top-side up. Maria helped us consider all our birth options along with the doctors, who also were working with us to help get the baby turned around. Once again, we decided that going to the hospital and having a C-section birth was the best and safest route for the baby and me. Maria worked with my husband and me to prepare for the C-section birth, stayed with us in the hospital as I labored for seven hours and then was with us in the operating room. She stayed by my side during and after the delivery, which allowed my husband to be with the baby immediately after she was born and stay with her until I was in recovery. Again, even though I ended up having a second C-section, I felt that working with a knowledgeable and supportive midwife like Maria was the key to successful birth of our daughter.

After the birth of both my children, the ongoing support and knowledge that both midwives brought to me and my family during their postpartum home visits was invaluable. I found great comfort and support in having my midwife, who had worked with me for several months, come to my home as I recovered from a C-section birth and worked with my baby to nurse successfully.

I am looking forward to working with a midwife again when the time comes to have my third child.

—*Proud mommie Meikle*

Birth Statistics From The National Center For Health Statistics

The following are the most recent facts and figures available regarding birth and birth rate in the United States. These facts are taken from the details included on birth certificates. It is important to note that some facts may be under-reported on birth certificates.

Number of Births

There were 4,025,933 births in the U.S. in 2001, 1% fewer than the previous year. This marks the first decline in the number of births, following three consecutive years of increases. The crude birth rate for 2001 was 14.1 births per 1,000 total population, compared with 14.4 in 2000. The 2001 rate was 16% lower than in 1990 and a record low for the nation. The first birth rate declined in 2001 to 26.6 births per 1,000 women aged 15-44 years. The tendency of women to postpone childbearing continued; the median age at first birth rose from 24.6 to 24.8 years, and has risen from 22.1 years since 1970.

Fertility Rate

The general fertility rate, which relates births to the number of women in the childbearing ages, was 65.3 per 1,000 women aged 15-44 years in 2001, about 1% lower than in 2000, and 8% below the 1990 level.

Age of Mother

<u>Women in their twenties</u>: Birth rates for women in their twenties declined in 2001. The rate for women aged 20-24 years dropped 2%. The rate for 25-29 year-olds was also down very slightly.

<u>Women in their thirties</u>: Birth rates for women in their thirties increased 1-2%: **30-34 years** increased 1% and **35-39 years** increased 2%. Rates for these age groups have risen 20 and 30 percent, respectively, over the last decade.

<u>Women in their forties</u>: Births to women in this group increased to 8.1 per 1,000, matching the previous high in 1970.

<u>Women 50 years old and over</u>: Because of increases in fertility-enhancing therapies, greater numbers of women are giving birth at age 50 and older. In 1999, 174 births were reported to women aged 50-54 years.

AGE OF FATHER

The birth rate per 1,000 men aged 15-54 years was 50.6 in 2001, a decrease of 2% from 2000. During the first half of the 1990's, the overall birth rate for men declined 11%, but since 1996, this rate has fluctuated little, hovering around 51.

MATERNAL LIFESTYLE AND HEALTH CHARACTERISTICS

Maternal weight gain during pregnancy influences pregnancy outcome. Inadequate maternal weight gain has been associated with an increased risk of intrauterine growth retardation, shortened period of gestation, low birth weight, and perinatal mortality. High weight gain during pregnancy has been linked with an elevated risk of a large-for-gestational-age (LGA) infant, cesarean delivery, and long-term maternal weight retention. In 1990 the Institute of Medicine (IOM) published guidelines for weight gain during pregnancy for singleton gestation. The guidelines recommend that women who are underweight gain 28-40 pounds, those who are of normal weight gain 25-35 pounds, and those who are overweight gain 15-25 pounds. However, it recommended that weight gain goals be tailored to individual needs. In 2001, almost one in three women gained outside the IOM guidelines.

MEDICAL RISK FACTORS

Medical risk factors during pregnancy can contribute to serious complications and maternal and infant morbidity and mortality, particularly if not treated properly. In 2001, the most frequently reported medical risk factors were pregnancy-associated hypertension, diabetes and anemia. These have been the most frequently reported risk factors since these data have been available from birth certificates. Pregnancy-associated hypertension declined slightly in 2001 for the first time in over a decade after rising steadily since 1990. Rates for diabetes and anemia have also risen about 40% over this time period.

PRENATAL CARE

Women were more likely to have timely **prenatal care** in 2001. Timely care has risen 10 percent since 1990.

OBSTETRIC PROCEDURES

Six specific obstetric procedures are listed on the birth certificate. Of these, **electronic fetal monitoring** (EFM) was the most frequently reported in 2001, as in earlier years. More than 67% of women who had live births in 2001 received **ultrasound**. The use of this procedure has increased steadily since 1989. The rate of **induction** of labor for 2001 was more than double the 1989 level. Between 1989 (the first year these data were reported on birth certificates) and 2000, the rate of induction rose every year for all gestational ages, including preterm delivery. However, for 2001, the induction rate rose only for gestational ages of 37 weeks or more. Recent articles on the indications for induction suggest that the growth in the induction rate may be due, in part, to an increase in elective inductions (inductions with no medical or obstetric indication). The **rate of stimulation of labor** was 17.5%; this figure has fluctuated only slightly since 1997. However, the 2001 rate is almost two-thirds higher than the 1989 level. The overall rate for **tocolysis,** the use of agents that decrease uterine activity for the management of preterm labor has been fairly stable since 1996. In 2001, the overall rate for **amniocentesis** decreased to 2.2 percent of births in 2001. This change may reflect the use of screening tests that are noninvasive (*e.g.* ultrasound and measurement of serum markers) in lieu of amniocentesis.

COMPLICATIONS OF LABOR AND DELIVERY

Of the 15 complications of labor and/or delivery reported on the birth certificate, the five most frequently reported for 2001 were meconium moderate/heavy, fetal distress, breech/malpresentation, dysfunctional labor, and premature rupture of membrane (PROM).

ATTENDANT AT BIRTH AND PLACE OF DELIVERY

In 2001, the trends in attendant at birth and place of delivery observed for recent years continued. The percent of all births delivered by physicians in hospitals continued to decline slowly but steadily, to 91.3% of all births compared to 98.7% in 1975. The percent of births attended by midwives has increased steadily since 1975. Midwifery education and hence practice have grown over the past decade. A recent report found that nearly all of the increase in midwife-attended births was for those in hospitals. Almost 95% of all midwife-attended births in 2001 were by certified nurse midwives (CNMs). Ninety-nine percent of births in 2001 were delivered in hospitals, essentially unchanged for the last several decades. The majority of out-of-hospital births were in a residence (65%); 28% were in a freestanding birthing center. This level has been fairly stable since 1989.

METHOD OF DELIVERY

In 2001, nearly one in four live births were delivered by cesarean section. The rate of cesarean delivery climbed to 24.4% of all births, a 7% rise from 2000. This rate fell each year between 1989 and 1996, but has risen each year since 1996, by a total of 18%, and is now the highest reported since these data became available from birth certificates. This rise in the total rate is due to both the growth in the primary cesarean rate and a steep decrease in the rate of vaginal birth after cesarean delivery. As might be anticipated, coinciding with the rise in the cesarean delivery rate, the percent of births delivered by either forceps or vacuum extraction decreased between 2000 and 2001, from 7.0% to 6.3%.

INFANT HEALTH CHARACTERISTICS

PERIOD OF GESTATION

The **percent of infants born preterm**, or at less than 37 weeks of gestation, increased to 11.9% for 2001, the highest level in at least two decades. The preterm birth rate has risen 27% since 1981. The upward trend in preterm births over the past 20 years has been influenced in part by the rise in the multiple birth rate (preterm rates are much higher among multiple births than among singletons), and by the increase in preterm multiple deliveries. For the current year, 6.9% of births were delivered **post-term**, or at 42 or more weeks of gestation. This is more than a one-third decline from the level reported in 1990.

BIRTH WEIGHT

The low birth weight rate (LBW), less than five and a half pounds, was 7.7% for 2001, up slightly from 7.6% for 2000 the highest level recorded since the early 1970s. The percent of very low birth weight (VLBW), less than three and one fourth pounds, has been fairly stable since 1997. The percent of higher birth weight or macrosomic births, or at least eight pounds, 14 ounces, was down markedly between 2000 and 2001, from 9.9 to 9.4%. The proportion of higher birth weight infants has generally trended downward after peaking at around 11% in the 1980s. The mean birth weight for singleton births for 2001 was seven pounds, six ounces.

Multiple Births

The twin birth rate rose 3% to 30.1 per 1,000 in 2001. The twinning rate has risen 33% since 1990, and 59% since 1980. Following a two-year decline, the rate of triplet and other higher order multiple births rose 3% to 185.6 per 100,000, but remained lower than the 1998 peak. The triplet/and birth rate has climbed more than 400 percent since 1980.

National Center for Health Statistics. 2002-3.

Questions to Ask in Planning Your Child's Birth

from the Coalition for Improving Maternity Services

Where is the Best Place to Start?

In 1996, after two years of meetings, approximately 25 prominent childbirth education organizations and 30 midwives, physicians, nurses, childbirth educators, labor support providers, lactation consultants, postpartum care providers, and consumer advocates created the Mother-Friendly Childbirth Initiative. The Coalition for Improving Maternity Services (CIMS—pronounced "Kims") has grown to represent more then 90,000 birth professionals.

The Initiative is an evidence-based document, which provides guidelines for identifying and designating mother-friendly birth sites including hospitals, birth centers, and home-birth services. The Initiative outlines ten steps for mother-friendly care (defined below), and includes as a requirement that mother-friendly birthing services also qualify as "baby-friendly" according to the World Health Organization's guidelines.

Having a Baby? Ten Questions to Ask

First, you should learn as much as you can about all your choices. There are many different ways of caring for a mother and her baby during labor and birth. Birthing care that is better and healthier for mothers and babies is called "mother-friendly." Some birthplaces or settings are more mother-friendly than others. A group of experts in birthing care came up with this list of ten things to look for and ask about. Medical research supports all of these things. These are also the best ways to be mother-friendly. When you are deciding where to have your baby, you'll probably be choosing from different places such as birth center, hospital, or home birth service.

Here's what you should expect, and ask for, in your birth experience. Be sure to find out how the people you talk with handle these ten issues about caring for you and your baby. You may want to ask the following questions to help you learn more.

1. WHO CAN BE WITH ME DURING LABOR AND BIRTH?

Mother-friendly birth centers, hospitals, and home birth centers will let a birthing mother decide whom she wants to have with her during the birth. This includes fathers, partners, children, other family members, or friends. They will also let a birthing mother have with her a person who has special training in helping women cope with labor and birth. This person is called a doula or labor support person. She never leaves the birthing mother alone. She encourages her, comforts her, and helps her understand what's happening to her. They will also have midwives as part of their staff so that a birthing mother can have a midwife with her if she wants to.

2. WHAT HAPPENS DURING A NORMAL LABOR AND BIRTH IN YOUR SETTING?

If they give mother-friendly care, they will tell you they handle every part of the birthing process. For example, how often do they give the mother a drug to speed up the birth? Or do they let labor and birth usually happen on its own timing?

They will also tell you how often they do certain procedures. For example, they will have a record of the percentage of C-sections (cesarean births) they do every year. If the number is too high, you'll want to consider having your baby in another place or with another doctor or midwife. (See later section for statistics regarding C-section.)

Here are some numbers we recommend you ask about:
- They should not use oxytocin (a drug) to start or speed up labor for more than one in ten women (10%).
- They should not do an episiotomy (ee-pee-zee-AH-tummy) on more than one in five women (20%). They should be trying to bring that number down. (An episiotomy is a cut in the opening to the vagina to make it larger for birth. It is not necessary most of the time.)

- They should not do C-sections on more than one in ten women (10%) if it's a community hospital. The rate should be 15% or less in hospitals that care for many high-risk mothers and babies. A C-section is a major operation in which a doctor cuts through the mother's stomach into her womb and removes the baby through the opening. Mothers who have a C-section can often have future babies normally. Look for a birthplace in which six out of ten women (60%) or more of the mothers who have had C-sections go on to have other babies through the birth canal.

3. How do you allow for differences in culture and beliefs?

Mother-friendly birth centers, hospitals, and home birth services are sensitive to the mother's culture. They know that mothers and fathers have differing beliefs, values and customs.

For example, you may have a custom that only women may be with you during labor and birth. Or, perhaps your beliefs include a religious ritual to be done after birth. There are many other examples that may be important to you. If the place and the people are mother-friendly, they will support you in doing what you want to do. Before labor starts tell your doctor or midwife special things you want.

4. Can I walk and move around during labor? What position do you suggest for birth?

In mother-friendly settings, you can walk around and move as you choose during labor. You can choose the positions that are most comfortable and work best for you during labor and birth. (There may be a medical reason for you to be in a certain position.) Mother-friendly settings almost never put a woman flat on her back with her legs in stirrups for the birth.

5. How do you make sure ... my nurse, doctor, midwife or agency work together? Can you help me find people or agencies in my community who can help me before and after the baby is born?

Mother-friendly places will have a specific plan for keeping in touch with the other people who are caring for you. They will talk to others who give you birth care. They will help you find people or agencies in your community to help you. For example, they may put you in touch with someone who can help you with breast-feeding.

6. What things do you normally do to a woman in labor?

Experts say some methods of care during labor and birth are better and healthier for mothers and babies. Medical research shows us which methods of care are better and healthier. Mother-friendly settings only use methods that have been proven to be best by scientific evidence.

Sometimes birth centers, hospitals, and home birth services use methods that are not proven to be best for the mother or the baby. For example, research has shown it's not usually not helpful to break the bag of waters.

Here is a list of things we recommend you ask about that do not help and may hurt healthy mothers and babies. They are not proven to be best for mother or baby and are not mother-friendly.
- They should not keep track of the baby's heart rate at all times with a machine (called an electronic fetal monitor). Instead it is best to have your nurse or midwife listen to the baby's heart from time to time.
- They should not break your bag of waters early in labor.
- They should not use an IV (a needle put into your vein to give you fluids).
- They should not tell you that you can't eat or drink during labor.
- They should not shave you.
- They should not give you an enema.

A birth center, hospital, or home birth service that does these things for most mothers is not mother-friendly. Remember, these should not be used without a special medical reason.

7. How do you help mothers stay as comfortable as they can be? Besides drugs, how do you help mothers relieve pain?

The people who care for you should know how to help you cope with labor. They should know about ways of dealing with pain that don't use drugs. They should suggest such things as changing your position, relaxing in a warm bath, having a massage, and using music. These are called comfort measures.

Comfort measures help you handle labor more easily and help you feel more in control. The people who care for you will not try to persuade you to use a drug for pain unless you need it to take care of a special medical problem. All drugs affect the baby.

8. What if my baby is born early or has special problems?

Mother-friendly places and people will encourage mothers and families to touch, hold, breast-feed, and care for their babies as much as they can. They will encourage this even if your baby is born early or has a medical problem at birth. (However, there may be a special medical reason you shouldn't hold and care for your baby.)

9. DO YOU CIRCUMCISE BABY BOYS?

Medical research does not show a need to circumcise baby boys. It is painful and risky. Mother-friendly birth places discourage circumcision unless it is for religious reasons.

10. HOW DO YOU HELP MOTHERS WHO WANT TO BREAST-FEED?

The World Health Organization made this list of ways birth services support breast-feeding.
- They tell all pregnant mothers why and how to breast-feed.
- They help you start breast-feeding within one hour after your baby is born.
- They show you how to breast-feed. And they show you how to keep your milk coming in even if you have to be away from your baby for work or other reasons.
- Newborns should only have breast milk. (However, there may be a medical reason they cannot have it right away.)
- They encourage you and the baby to stay together all day and all night. This is called "rooming-in."
- They encourage you to feed your baby whenever he or she wants to nurse, rather than at certain times.
- They should not give pacifiers ("dummies" or "soothers") to breast-fed babies.
- They encourage you to join a group of mothers who breast-feed.
- They tell you how to contact a group near you.
- They have a written policy on breast-feeding. All the employees know about and use the ideas in the policy.
- They teach employees the skills they need to carry out these steps.

Reprinted with the permission of the Coalition for Improving Maternity Services (CIMS). They may be contacted at:
CIMS National Office
P.O. Box 2346
Ponte Vedra Beach, Florida 32004
1-888-282-CIMS
904-285-1613, Fax: 904-285-2120, www.motherfriendly.org,
info@motherfriendly.org

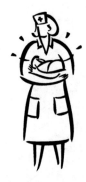

Part Two: Choices of Birth Professionals

Choices of Birth Professionals

PHYSICIANS
by Regula E. Burki, MD, FACOG

CHOICES OF PHYSICIANS WHO DELIVER BABIES

In the 21st century, we have several options when it comes to obstetrical care. Think about your priorities in pregnancy and childbirth, so you can choose someone who shares your birth philosophy. Know what your backup arrangements are should your pregnancy or delivery become more complicated than you expected. Here are some basic definitions of the types of caregivers available. They vary as professionals and as individuals in training, style, experience and competence.

Three types of physicians provide pregnancy and birthing care:

- Family Practitioners
- Obstetricians and
- Maternal-Fetal Medicine Specialists/Perinatologists

They all have earned an undergraduate college degree and completed four years of medical school, followed by three to four years of residency training in a specialty program accredited by the Accreditation Council for Graduate Medical Education (ACGME). Perinatologists complete an additional two to three years of training after their OB/GYN residency.

General practitioners are physicians who have completed four years of medical school and one year of internship, but have not received any residency training before entering practice. They are not eligible for any board certification examinations and rarely deliver babies.

DOCTORS OF OSTEOPATHIC MEDICINE (DOs)

DOs complete their postgraduate training at a College of Osteopathic medicine instead of a medical school. They can receive the same type of residency and fellowship training as MDs. DOs delivered 4.3% of all babies delivered by a physician in 2001.

Obstetrician/Gynecologist (OB/GYN)

An obstetrician is a physician who specializes in pregnancy and childbirth, as well as in gynecology: women-specific medicine. An OB/GYN receives four years of residency training in obstetrics and gynecology. He or she is then eligible to take both a written and oral board certification exam given by a panel of experts. The oral exam includes an extensive review of the management of both obstetrical and gynecological cases treated the year prior to the oral examination. Only OB/GYNs who are certified by the American Board of Obstetrics and Gynecology can become Fellows of the American College of Obstetricians and Gynecologists and place the letters FACOG after their name. A Junior ACOG Fellow is an OB/GYN who has met all criteria of ACOG membership, but not yet completed both board certification examinations. Obstetricians generally deliver in hospitals and birthing centers.

Family Physician

A family practitioner is trained in all aspects of family medicine, including the management of uncomplicated pregnancy, labor and delivery. A family practitioner completes three years of residency training. After passing a written certification examination administered by the American Board of Family Practice he or she is eligible for membership in the American Academy of Family Physicians and may place the letters AAFP after his or her name.

In rural areas, where there are no obstetricians available, they sometimes also perform cesarean sections. In urban areas, the majority of family physicians no longer provide obstetrical care, because of prohibitive professional liability premiums and because the courts hold them to the same standard of care as the specialists.

Family physicians deliver at hospitals and birthing centers and must have a consultative arrangement with an obstetrician as back-up for complications as a condition of their privileges at these institutions. Depending on the degree of risk and the availability of specialists, family practitioners refer more complicated pregnancies to the care of either an obstetrician or a perinatologist.

Maternal-Fetal Medicine Specialist/Perinatologist

MFM specialists are obstetrician/gynecologists who have completed two to three years of additional formal education and clinical experience within an American Board of Obstetrics and Gynecology (ABOG) approved Maternal-Fetal Medicine Fellowship Program. After board certification in obstetrics and gynecology and completing an accredited fellowship program, an MFM specialist must take a second set of written and oral certification exams in order to become board-certified in the subspecialty of Maternal Fetal Medicine.

Only MFM specialists who have passed the subspecialty board exams can become full members of the Society of Maternal Fetal Medicine. Members of the Society have advanced knowledge of the obstetrical, medical, genetic, and surgical complications of pregnancy and their effects on both the mother and fetus. The society has around 2,000 world wide members.

High-risk pregnancies are referred by both family practitioners and obstetricians to MFM specialists, who usually practice at a university medical center or a tertiary care center equipped with a neonatal intensive care unit.

Questions to Ask Your Physician

Are you a preferred provider under my insurance plan?

Before you make an appointment, make sure the physician is listed with your insurance carrier as a preferred provider.

At which hospitals do you deliver?

Which of these hospitals are on your insurance plan? What emergency facilities do they have? How is the nursery equipped? Do they have a neonatal specialist on call? Is that specialist staying in house? How far is the hospital from your house? How long does it take to get there during rush hour?

You may also want to tour the facility and look at their labor and delivery rooms. Do they have birthing rooms, or will you be moved to a delivery room to deliver? (That could mean a frantic trip through the hallways as you are about to give birth and is far from pleasant and not particularly safe.) What are the hospital's regulations regarding visitors during labor?

Are you board-certified?

The easiest way to find that out is to look for the letters AAFP (American Academy of Family Physicians) or FACOG (Fellow of the American College of Obstetricians and Gynecologists) behind your doctor's name. This assures that the doctor is board-certified and a member in good standing in the professional organization of his or her specialty.

Both organizations require periodic recertification exams, as well as documentation of a set number of hours of continuing medical education. To be admitted to the board certification examinations, the doctor must have either graduated from an accredited U.S. medical school and residency program or, as a foreign medical graduate, have taken a series of qualifying exams.

Alternatively, you can call the medical staff office of the hospital where you plan to deliver. Most hospitals nowadays require board certification as a condition of admission privileges. Older physicians may have been grandfathered in without board certification.

WHAT COVERAGE ARRANGEMENTS DO YOU HAVE?

You should ask the doctor or the office nurse this question directly. Some doctors deliver all their patients during the week and share call only on weekends and holidays. Other doctors have call arrangements with their colleagues that do not differentiate between weekdays and holidays. Will you get to meet the other doctors in the call group who might potentially deliver your baby?

WHO WILL BE ATTENDING ME DURING LABOR?

Some very busy doctors have their own nurses or midwives monitor their patients during labor. This system ensures that their patients are will taken care of and that the doctors are notified in time if there is a problem. Because of managed care and a severe nurse shortage in parts of the country, hospitals have cut back staff on labor and delivery floors resulting in the patient per nurse ratio often being too high. Your insurance may or may not cover the expense of a private attendant, but if you can afford it, she may be well worth it. On the other hand, your doctor may feel comfortable with the staffing ratio and quality and experience of the staff at the hospital, making this extra expense unnecessary.

HOW DO YOU FEEL ABOUT LABOR COACHES?

Depending on your personal support system, i.e., the father of your baby, your partner, sister, or friend, you may want to hire a labor coach. Does you doctor feel comfortable having a labor coach present? Does she have someone she often collaborates with? The last thing you want when you are having your baby is your coach and doctor arguing over the management of your labor!

How far do you live from the hospital?

Find out how far your doctor lives from the hospital, if she stays in the hospital (or at least in the office building next door) while you are in the late stages of labor, how many different hospitals the doctor is on call for at the same time, and what her track record is for showing up on time in an emergency.

This is not information to ask your doctor directly! Most doctors would be rather taken aback and offended by these kinds of questions and feel that you are likely to sue them. Given the current litigious environment in the U.S. this is not an unreasonable concern. Nevertheless, it might start your doctor-patient relationship on the wrong foot. On the other hand, they are important questions. The best way to get them answered is a first name only phone call to the labor and delivery floor of the hospital or the birthing center. Make sure to ask at the outset if they are swamped or not. They will be much more willing to chat with you if things are slow. Avoid calling during shift change.

Questions That Are Not Helpful or Relevant

What is your cesarean section rate?

The C-section rate depends very much on the population of women whose babies your doctor delivers and in no way reflects the doctor's competence. A high risk specialist, who takes care of pregnancies complicated by multiple fetuses, premature labor, toxemia, preexisting medical diseases and other obstetrical complications, will perform many more C-sections than an average obstetrician. Likewise, an obstetrician practicing at a hospital with a neonatal intensive care unit will attract higher risk patients and have a higher C-section rate than one practicing at a community hospital.

After several years of decline, the C-section rate is now increasing again. After publication of the true complication rates and the often fatal nature of these complications, women and their doctors are no longer (monetarily) coerced by their health insurance into vaginal births after a previous C-section (VBAC).

Have you been sued?

Recent studies show that 70-80% of obstetricians have been sued at least once. Furthermore, the risk of being sued varies widely by geographical location, *i.e.*, a doctor in Wyoming is five times more likely to be sued than a doctor in Alabama. Even finding out whether a case was fought and won by a doctor or settled does not tell you much. Until recently many doctors were forced by their liability carriers to settle cases, because it was cheaper for the insurer to pay a settlement than to pay lawyers to fight it in court. Only about 10 to 15 cents per dollar awarded in a malpractice suit actually go to the patient. However, large numbers of lawsuits per doctor do correlate with training at inferior institutions and lack of board certification. Verifying your doctor's training is still the best predictor of competence.

Dr. Regula E. Burki is an OB/GYN and a Fellow of the American College of Obstetricians and Gynecologists (ACOG). Prior to entering private practice she was a Clinical Fellow in Obstetrics and Gynecology at Harvard University and completed a residency in Obstetrics and Gynecology at Massachusetts General Hospital in Boston, where she served as chief resident. She is the current Chair of the Utah section of the American College of Obstetricians and Gynecologists and a diplomat of the American Board of Obstetrics and Gynecology. She maintains a private practice in gynecology in Salt Lake City, Utah. The views Dr. Burki expresses in this book are her personal views and not necessarily those of ACOG.

Regula E. Burki, MD, FACOG
1250 East 3900 South, Suite 205
Salt Lake City, Utah 84124
phone: 801-262-2788; fax: 801-262-3684
reburki@msn.com

HOW TO SELECT A DOCTOR, COMMUNICATE WITH A DOCTOR AND KNOW WHEN TO CHANGE DOCTORS

by Regula E. Burki, MD, FACOG

It is very hard for an ordinary person to select a physician without "inside" information because a good bedside manner in no way guarantees competence.

Most hospitals have a physician referral service that will answer questions about training, years in practice, board certification, as well as what insurance plans a given physician belongs to. The State Medical Associations provide a similar service.

If you have a doctor you trust, ask her what specialists she used for her family. If your doctor refers you to someone, you can generally assume that you are being referred to a competent physician. It reflects badly on a physician to refer a patient to someone less than competent. In addition, a physician is legally liable for knowingly referring a patient to substandard care.

It is also often useful to check with hospital nurses. For instance, if you are pregnant in a new city, you could call the head nurse on labor and delivery in the closest hospital and ask her whom she would pick for herself. She will know which doctors arrive promptly and are able to handle emergencies. When my pediatrician suggested a surgeon for my son, I cross-checked with the head nurse in the operating room.

Polling your friends is an obvious way to find a doctor. They can give you information about office staff, waiting time, a doctor's willingness to answer questions and return phone calls, ability to talk in nonmedical terms that patients can understand, etc.

Also take into consideration whether you are selecting a physician for ongoing care or for a one-time service. You will want the technically best heart surgeon, for instance, but the cardiologist who will manage your heart medications for the rest of your life should also have a well organized office with minimal waiting time, be willing to return your calls, etc.

Personally, I would give up a medically excellent doctor if I repeatedly had to wait more than 20 minutes for an appointment, if the physician were patronizing or unwilling to answer all my questions in an easy to understand manner, if I were not allowed to talk to the doctor and the nurse was unable to answer questions to my satisfaction, if I were unable to reach the doctor or someone covering for emergencies when the office was closed, and—of course—if there was even a hint of sexual impropriety. For the last transgression I would immediately report the doctor to the Medical Association and Licensing Board. I would bring unhelpful or inefficient office personnel to the doctor's attention, but that reason alone would not make me change doctors.

MIDWIVES

from the Midwives' Alliance of North America

What is a Midwife?

A midwife is a trained professional who offers expert care, education, counseling and support to a woman and her newborn during the childbearing cycle. The midwife works with each woman and her family to identify their unique physical, social, and emotional needs. In addition, many midwives provide well-woman gynecological care and family planning services. Midwives know how to watch for and identify potential or actual complications, and they can provide emergency treatment until additional assistance is available.

What do Midwives do?

Midwives offer:
- prenatal care that promotes informed decision making;
- choice of birth place;
- education and counseling;
- labor support, birth and postpartum care;
- support for bonding;
- examination and evaluation of the newborn;
- breast-feeding support;
- counseling in early parenting; and
- well-woman care.

The History of Midwifery

Midwife means "with woman." Traditionally, women have attended and assisted other women during labor and birth. As modern medicine emerged in the Western World, birth was sacrificed to the medical model. Due to the predominance of men in the medical field, men became the birth practitioners. Having never given birth themselves, they did not possess any of the experiences or knowledge of a woman. Childbirth became viewed as an illness or condition. This resulted in many unnecessary medical techniques and interventions being introduced.

During the 1960s and 1970s, midwifery once again became an important force. More families were considering homebirth and, along with this, the natural choice of a midwife. Midwifery has been growing steadily ever since. Midwives are becoming more and more involved with birthing families and have been instrumental in redefining birth as a natural event in the life of a woman.

When a woman gives birth with the help of a midwife, she is given back control of the entire experience. She, her partner, and her family are all a part of this experience.

MIDWIFERY IN THE UNITED STATES

Midwives are recognized throughout the world as the most appropriate maternity care provider for most women. Midwifery licensure and scope of practice in the United States are regulated by individual state laws. Four categories of professional midwives are recognized in the United States:

DIRECT-ENTRY MIDWIVES

"Direct-entry" midwives, who are licensed in some states, are not required to become nurses before training to be midwives. The Midwifery Education and Accreditation Council (MEAC) is currently accrediting direct-entry midwifery educational programs and apprenticeships in the United States. Direct-entry midwives' legal status varies according to state, and they practice most often in birth centers and homes.

CERTIFIED PROFESSIONAL MIDWIVES (CPMs)

Certified Professional Midwives may gain their midwifery education through a variety of routes. They must have their midwifery skills and experience evaluated through the North American Registry of Midwives (NARM) certification process and pass the NARM Written Examination and Skills Assessment. The legal status of these nationally credentialed direct-entry midwives varies from state to state. In some states where they are also individually licensed, midwives' services are reimbursable through Medicaid and private insurance carriers.

CERTIFIED NURSE-MIDWIVES (CNMs)

Certified Nurse-Midwives are educated in both nursing and midwifery. To earn the CNM credential, individuals must graduate from an education program that has been accredited by the American College of Nurse-Midwives (ACNM) Division of Accreditation. Graduates, who have earned at least a bachelor's degree, must then pass the ACNM Certification Council, Inc. (ACC) exam. CNMs are licensed to practice in 50 states and provide primary health care to women, with a focus on maternity and gynecological services. CNMs practice most often in hospitals and birth centers.

Certified Midwives (CMs)
Certified Midwives are also graduates of ACNM accredited education programs who have at least a bachelor's degree and have passed the ACC certification exam. These individuals, who are prepared to provide the same scope of service as their CNM colleagues, do not have to be registered nurses.

Midwifery Care is Cost-effective
Midwifery fees are typically one-third less than fees for comparable services provided by physicians; midwifery care saves money without sacrificing quality or safety.

Midwives Provide Personalized Care
Women want more than technological care during pregnancy and birth. Midwives encourage participation by family members and provide continuous support during labor and birth. Midwives trust the birth process and affirm each individual woman's ability to give birth.

Midwives Encourage Informed Choices
Midwives encourage women and their families to take an active part in their own health care. Pregnancy is an ideal time to educate mothers about nutrition, healthful birth practices, breast-feeding, and infant care.

Midwifery Care Offers Choice of Birth Places
Midwives practice in homes, birth centers and hospitals. Midwives support the right of parents to choose the birth place that best suits their needs.

Midwifery Care Makes a Difference
Midwives worldwide have an excellent record of safety with numerous studies associating midwifery care with excellent outcomes. In five nations with the world's lowest infant mortality and lowest rates of technological intervention, midwives attend 70 percent of all births without a physician in the birth room.

For more information contact:
Midwives Alliance of North America (MANA)
4805 Lawrenceville Hwy., Suite 116-279
Lilburn, GA 30047

1-888-923-MANA (6262)
http://www.mana.org

North American Registry of Midwives (NARM)
5257 Rosestone Dr.
Lilburn, GA 30047
1-888-84-birth (24784)
http://www.narm.org

Midwifery Education and Accreditation Council (MEAC)
220 W. Birch
Flagstaff, AZ 86001
928-214-0997
http://www.meacschools.org

American College of Nurse-Midwives (ACNM)
818 Connecticut Ave. NW #900
Washington, DC 20006
202-728-9860
http://www.midwife.org

Questions To Ask A Midwife:

- What is your training and experience?
- Where did you train; how long have you been a midwife; and how many births have you attended?
- What is your basic philosophy of childbirth?
- Are you a licensed lay midwife or a certified nurse-midwife?
- Do you belong to any midwifery organizations, attend conferences and workshops, and subscribe to professional journals?
- Do you practice with other midwives? Will one of them provide backup if you are not available? Will I have an opportunity to meet that person?
- Are you easily contacted when needed? Do you have a pager or cellular phone?
- Do you have obstetrical backup? Ask for that person's name and phone number.
- What do you do in situations when complications arise? How do you organize a transfer to a hospital? Under what conditions would you organize a transfer? Would you still be involved in the birth?
- Describe the extent of your prenatal and postnatal care.

- Do you perform episiotomies? Under what circumstances? When tearing occurs, are you trained in suturing the perineum?
- What equipment will you bring to the birth?
- Are you certified in neonatal resuscitation? What resuscitation equipment do you have?
- How do you deal with newborn problems and emergencies? What is your experience in this area?
- Can you provide references from mothers you recently attended?
- Can you provide references from another midwife?
- What are your fees and will insurance cover your services?

It is very important that you are clear about what you expect from your potential midwife. Discuss your vision, expectations and any fears that you may have.

Prenatal Care, Labor, Birth and Postnatal Care with a Midwife

Prenatal Care

Prenatal visits are a time for the woman, family and midwife to get to know one another. Midwives include the family during prenatal care, inviting them to ask questions and listen to the baby's heartbeat. Intimate involvement of the family throughout the pregnancy allows for early bonding of the new family. As with any prenatal care, the midwife discusses nutrition, exercise and physical and emotional well-being. It is also their role to determine if any high-risk condition may exist. As midwives have varying levels of experience, some are more comfortable than others when handling a high risk situation. The midwife also oversees the healthy development of the fetus.

During the prenatal time, the midwife also helps the family prepare for the birth. It is important that all the family members involved know what to expect. A birth plan may be written to help clarify these expectations and may include the desires and wishes of the family members.

Labor and Birth

The midwife is called as soon as the mother goes into labor. She will provide the necessary support to both the mother and those present for the birth. The midwife is watchful for any complications or signs of distress in either the mom or the baby. Throughout labor, the midwife asks permission to perform any procedure and explains to the mom and family what she is doing and why. The birthing process is allowed to take its own course and set its own pace.

If complications arise, the midwife is trained to recognize the early stages of complications and to take the necessary action. The midwife and mother have had the opportunity to build a relationship, and this allows the mother to relax and put her faith in the midwife. This enhances the birth process. Labor and childbirth are a natural process and, unless distress to the mother or baby is indicated, there is no intervention through drugs or medical equipment. The mother, however, can at any time request intervention.

Postpartum Care

The midwife is still accessible to the mother after birth to provide information and support. This is of great importance, particularly to new moms who have questions or problems. The midwife will continue to check in on mother, baby and family up to about six weeks. However, this varies and should be clarified from the beginning.

Some information for Prenatal Care, Labor and Delivery and Postpartum Care provided by Midwifery Today, Inc.

Midwifery: The Art of Doing "Nothing" Well

by Nancy Sullivan, CNM, MS, FACNM

You might be surprised to learn that about 10% of all babies born in the United States today, up to 25% in some states, are delivered into the hands of a midwife. While it is the perception of many people that midwifery is as extinct as the dinosaur, the fact is that this very old and very new profession is alive and flourishing. Midwives are working, legally and with credentials, in every state in the union, in hospitals, birthing centers, and in the home. Why are so many parents opting to have their baby with a midwife?

Holly Powell Kennedy, a nurse-midwife and midwifery educator, studied "exemplary" midwives and their patients to try and learn what is unique and exemplary about the midwifery model of care. That is, what is different about the way that midwives provide care from the way that physicians provide care? She included both hospital-based, birth center, and home birth midwives in her study. The critical difference that emerged was the midwives' art of doing "nothing" well; that is, being present with the woman, being vigilant to assure that things were going well, but not intervening or using technology unless it was necessary. One woman summed it up by saying, "A large part of her providing the kind of care we wanted is what she didn't do . . . she didn't rush anything . . . she said to me, 'Your body knows what to do so just let it do it.'"

Some of the qualities that were strongly identified by women with midwifery care in Kennedy's study were belief in the normalcy of birth, exceptional clinical skills and judgment, and commitment to the health of women and families. The following terms were also strongly identified by women with the midwives who cared for them: calm, patient, confident, decisive, intelligent, mature, persistent, honest, compassionate, trustworthy, flexible, understanding and supportive, warm, nonjudgmental, gentle, nurturing, not focused on self, realistic, reassuring and soothing, possessing a generous and loving spirit, possessing a sense of humor, and being personable.

Midwives consider themselves to be the experts in normal childbirth. In Europe, midwives provide the majority of maternity care. Midwifery care leads to excellent outcomes; the infant mortality rate is lower in those countries that rely on midwives to care for most pregnant women, such as Holland and the Scandinavian countries. In our country, midwives were common until the first decades of the twentieth century, when physicians decided that obstetrics should become a medical specialty and that birth should take place in the hospital. The women who had been cared for in their homes by midwives were considered potential "training material" for medical students, and midwives were considered competition. Consequently, even though there were no statistics to show that midwives' care resulted in worse outcomes, midwifery was made illegal in many states, and the number of practicing midwives dwindled. This situation endured until the sixties and seventies, when two very separate trends contributed to a renaissance of midwifery. First, there was a "physician shortage," particularly when it came to caring for poor and uninsured women. Nurse-midwives, trained as public health nurses and given additional education as midwives, were recruited to care for poor women in under-served rural and inner-city communities. Second, the state of childbirth in the hospital had become so cold, so impersonal, and so "medicalized" that consumers began to rebel and seek a different form of care. "Lay" midwives, at first with little or no formal education, started assisting their friends and communities in giving birth at home.

Two types of professional midwives developed from these early prototypes. Certified nurse-midwives (CNMs) and certified midwives

(CMs) are educated in programs accredited by the American College of Nurse-Midwives and certified by the ACNM Certification Council. They are licensed in all fifty states. Although certified nurse-midwives continue to practice for the most part in the hospital setting and to a lesser extent in birth centers and the home, they strive to maintain the midwifery philosophy of care. Nonetheless, for some women, having a midwife-attended birth in the hospital is the perfect solution, since there is the option of high-tech procedures if they are needed. These might include epidural anesthesia, electronic monitoring, and intravenous medications. In addition, the midwife always has consultation and referral with an obstetrician readily available for complicated labors and possible operative deliveries.

Home-birth midwives, educated in formal midwifery schools accredited by the Midwifery Education and Accreditation Council or in apprenticeships, may be certified as Certified Professional Midwives (CPMs) by the North American Registry of Midwives. They practice legally in most states. Home-birth midwives, as well as midwives who practice in birth centers, should have strict criteria for women who are appropriate to deliver outside the hospital. They should have a plan for obstetric referral and hospital transfer if a problem should arise. For women who are low-risk and desire a home or birth-center birth, these options are safe and provide a level of comfort, familiarity, and intimacy for the family that is not possible in a hospital.

Midwives spend time with women, both during the prenatal visits and during labor. They expect questions. They encourage the women in their care to seek information and to come to their births as knowledgeable as possible, since knowledge is power. Nonetheless, they also encourage an attitude of flexibility, since every woman and every birth is unique and cannot be predicted. Midwives, like physicians, measure bellies, listen to baby heart rates, ask for urine samples and order ultrasounds, but they are interested in more than the physical progress of a woman's pregnancy and labor. They know that relationships and support systems, emotional and social stressors, spiritual beliefs, the childbirth experiences of their mothers, sisters and friends, and many other factors contribute to a woman's chances for a successful birth. They are concerned with good nutrition for a healthy baby and with exercise to optimize chances that the baby will come down the birth canal the right way. They are open to complementary treatments such as acupuncture, hypnotherapy, water birth, and massage. Above all, they believe that birth is a normal, physiological process that proceeds in the best way if left alone. Of course, there are situations in which pregnancy, labor, and birth are not normal. The midwife is trained to identify these cases and treat them if they are in her scope of practice, or consult or refer with her collaborating physician if necessary.

Midwifery care is supported by research. Many of the strategies used by midwives are supported by the Cochrane Collaboration, a systematic review of the research evidence about the effects of care given to women during pregnancy and childbirth. The Coalition for Improving Maternity Services, a group of individuals and national organizations with concern for the care and well-being of mothers, babies, and families offers an excellent document, "Having a Baby? Ten Questions to Ask" [reprinted in this book on page 44 which will get you started thinking about your choices for childbirth and reassure you that midwifery care is based on sound principles derived from scientific research, as well as on an art that has been passed down from our foremothers. This evidence-based mother-, baby-, and family-friendly model focuses on prevention and wellness, and emphasizes the midwife as the primary provider of maternity care. Another document to get you started thinking about your birth is the "Statement of the Rights of Childbearing Women," from the Maternity Center Association.

How can you find a midwife in your community? You can start by asking friends who have used a midwife for their birth. If none have, check the yellow pages under "Midwife" or call your local hospital and ask if they can recommend a midwife. There are several online directories of midwives, listed below. When you contact a midwife, ask to meet with her (or him; there are male midwives, too). Ask how she was trained or educated, what credentials she has, and how many births she has attended. Ask about her philosophy of care. Ask how she provides obstetric back-up in the case of complications. Ask her the "Ten Questions" mentioned above. Ask if she supports the "Statement of the Rights of Childbearing Women" published by the Maternity Center Association.

Midwifery care is not for everyone. If you have a chronic medical problem, such as diabetes, prior to becoming pregnant, or if your pregnancy becomes "high-risk" due to such problems as premature labor or hypertension, you need the specialized medical care offered by an obstetrician or perinatologist. If trying to safeguard the normalcy of your childbirth experience is not a priority, or if you want all the technology that modern medicine has to offer, you would probably be more comfortable with physician care. However, if you are intrigued by the possibility of making your birth a powerful and empowering experience, consider a midwife!

Information reprinted with the permission of Nancy Sullivan, CNM, MS, FACNM, a midwife and midwifery educator at Oregon Health Sciences University in Portland, Oregon. Since receiving her midwifery education at New York City's Columbia University in the early 1980s, she has helped more than 1,000 babies into the world. She is the founder and editor of www.midwifeinfo.com. Her daughter, Megan, is studying to be a midwife.

To contact Nancy Sullivan: Telephone 503-284-3771, FAX 413-513-3746, e-mail nancy@midwifeinfo.com, address 1915 NE Wasco Street, Portland OR 97232-1524

A Midwife's Tale

by Nancy Sullivan, CNM, MS, FACNM

How did I find the path to midwifery, why did I start down it, and what has kept me from wandering for over twenty years? The answer to the first two questions lies in my own birth experiences; as for the last, I have never considered looking back or changing direction, not even once. Oh, there have been times after several sleepless nights and disappointing births, head throbbing and unable to think, when I told myself that I was crazy. But I never thought of leaving midwifery.

I was introduced to midwifery when I was living with my family in France in the early '70s. I had eighteen-month-old twin daughters when we moved there. They were born in Houston, Texas, in 1969, at a time when "natural childbirth" was just coming into vogue. I had several friends in Houston who had gone through the childbirth education classes, and had tried to use some of what they had learned there during their labors. Most of them were unsuccessful—their husbands weren't allowed in the labor room, much less the delivery room; cameras were a no-no; either "twilight sleep" or a type of spinal anesthesia was required; and episiotomies were routinely cut. Rooming-in was unheard of, and breast-feeding was not encouraged. I was on bed rest for several months before my twins were born, so I couldn't attend the classes myself. I negotiated with my obstetrician—I wanted to be awake, but would accept a spinal if needed. Other than that, I didn't even know what to ask for.

I went through labor alone, in bed, without any medication or support. When I got to the delivery room, a caudal anesthetic was administered. I heard the doctor say, "Push!" and I tried with all my might to do so. "Oh," he said, "not you, Mrs. Sullivan. You can't feel anything." He was talking to the "fundal pressure" nurse who was pushing down on my belly with each contraction. My first daughter was born almost immediately afterward. After she emerged, my doctor reached up inside my uterus and found my second daughter's feet (she was lying sidewise), straightened her, and pulled her out—officially, three minutes later. I had an episiotomy, of course. Both babies were checked out and put into incubators. They were a little small, but otherwise very healthy. The nurse wheeled me into a little anteroom where my husband was waiting. She told us to get a good look at the babies, because we wouldn't be that close to them again until they were big enough to leave the hospital.

After I left the hospital, we were allowed to return once a day for fifteen minutes to look at the babies through a window. I had wanted to breast-feed, but that was not possible. I pumped and waited. After two weeks, we showed up one day to see the babies and were told they could go home. No one showed me how to bathe them, feed them, or care for them. The nurses just opened the door and passed them through to me, reminding us to complete the discharge paperwork.

In retrospect, I was very fortunate. A few years later, with a less experienced obstetrician, I would have almost certainly had a cesarean section because of the second twin's transverse position. I got to be awake and aware, but I didn't have a role in birthing my own babies. They had been "delivered" by the doctor and the nurse. Afterward, for the first two weeks of their lives, they seemed to belong to the hospital, not to me. I couldn't feed them, stroke them, cuddle them, talk to them. I found the whole experience unsettling and profoundly unsatisfying, and somewhere inside I knew there had to be a better way.

When I realized that I was pregnant again, five years later, I investigated my options in Paris and went to see an obstetrician at the American Hospital. Michel Odent [author of *Birth Reborn*] was working at Pithiviers, not far away, at that time, but I didn't know that. However, things went well. At the first visit, I asked the obstetrician if anesthesia and an episiotomy would be required for the birth. "Why, Madame?" he asked. "Do you expect to have a problem?" I asked him about childbirth education classes, and he said they were not common in France. However, he gave me the name of a midwife, a Mlle. Arnaud who did some teaching in her home. She was semi-retired after attending over 2,500 births in the public hospitals of Paris.

At my first appointment with Mlle. Arnaud, she told me that she would like to meet with me three or four times, and that she would come to the hospital to support me in labor. Also, she would come every day thereafter to help with breast-feeding. She was as good as her word. I had a short but very intense labor, and birthed a nine-pound thirteen ounce baby boy. I did have an episiotomy, not routine in France. I can still hear the doctor, the midwife, and the nurses all shouting, "Poussez, Madame!" and "Quelles epaules (what shoulders)!" as my son was being born. Shortly after, when I returned to my room, he was brought to me for breast-feeding and Mlle. Arnaud was there to assist. She came every day during the week I spent in the hospital.

During this time in France, several other things happened to push me toward the midwifery path. A bestselling book, *Journal d'une Sagefemme (Diary of a Midwife)*, appeared at all the bookstores. It was the autobiography of a young midwife from Martinique, Jacqueline Manicom, and told about her experiences as a midwife in the public hospitals of Paris alternately with her grandmother's story as a midwife in Martinique. I was totally captured by this account of midwifery, the first book in French that I managed to read cover to cover. When I wrote to a friend in the United States about my discovery of this oldest of professions, she sent me an article from one of the first issues of *Ms Magazine* about the renaissance of midwifery in America. It included some resources, including the address of the American College of Nurse-Midwives (ACNM). I immediately wrote and asked for a subscription to their journal. I applied to midwifery school in France, much to the consternation of the director, who had never had an American applicant before. However, before I could start the course of studies, my husband was transferred back to the states, and we found ourselves living in New York City.

I explored my options. "Lay" midwifery was illegal in New York. Nurse-midwifery required a nursing degree. As it turned out, we lived less than two blocks from Cornell University's medical school, and I entered their two-year nursing program in 1977. Graduating two years later, I worked for two years at Roosevelt Hospital on the postpartum floor and on labor and delivery. I chose Roosevelt because there were midwives there (the oldest private nurse-midwifery practice in the country, which is still active) and I wanted a recommendation to a midwifery program. I entered Columbia University's program in 1981 and graduated two years later. I will never forget the moment when I opened the envelope from the ACNM telling me that I had passed, that I was entitled to write "CNM" after my name.

Since that moment, I have never looked back. I have thought about the hardship that my passion for midwifery bestowed on my family; the years my son spent in nursery schools and daycare, after-school programs and summer camps; the important events in my family's lives that I missed or slept through; the change in my relationship with my husband that ultimately ended in divorce. Now that they are grown, my children are as proud of me as I am of them, and we are extremely close. One of my daughters has chosen to follow my path, and recently began her career as a midwife.

What has kept me on the path? I would say the answer is the many women I have assisted to birth their own babies and to feel good about and strengthened by their birth experiences. I have attended over 1,000 births, many memorable and wonderful, many sad and forgettable. I remember the first time that tears of joy didn't come to my eyes as the baby emerged, and later realized that this birth was the first I attended where the baby was not welcome, was not going to be received with love and attention.

Some births stand out. A young Vietnamese woman, 17 years old, who was alone in labor. Her labor stalled, and I spent hours helping her move and breathe. When she was exhausted, we got an epidural. When she was resting quietly through the night until it became apparent that she would need a cesarean section, she told me her story. Four years earlier, her family had sewn gold bars into her clothing and sent her away from Vietnam with the boat people, fearful that the family would not have a survivor and progenitor. She had wound up in Portland, stayed with distant relatives, and became pregnant after a short relationship with a schoolmate. I was so touched by this story, whose details I could only imagine, and by the calm determination of this young woman who had fulfilled her parents' wishes of providing them with a grandchild who would live in freedom. Several months later, she invited me to visit her and her son, Anthony. They lived in a subsidized apartment complex in the suburbs. It was empty except for a crib, a mattress on the floor, and a card table. It was immaculate. She fixed me Vietnamese iced coffee with sweet milk. She was planning to start college soon; Anthony would stay with relatives. She hoped someday to go back to Vietnam.

I also assisted a young career woman who was estranged from her mother and pregnant by her musician boyfriend who was uncertain about fatherhood and not completely supportive. When the baby failed to grow normally in mid-pregnancy, I ordered an ultrasound. Something was radically wrong, and further tests were done. The baby had a lethal genetic anomaly called triploidy—a whole extra set of genes. This terrible news alienated the boyfriend even more, and he didn't show up for appointments and broke other promises. However, when this woman went into labor, he was there. The mother was there, having flown all night from the east coast. Friends were there with candles, music, prayers, hugs. The labor was fast and easy because the baby was so small. I was worried that the baby would look strange, and to me she did. But to this mother, she was perfect, only small. She was named and baptized. She lived for half an hour, cradled in her mother's arms and greeted by her family and friends with prayers, poems, and songs of welcome and good-bye.

A perfect birth was a mother in her late thirties, with three young boys, pregnant for the last time and hoping for a daughter. She came to me because she had had "medical model" births the first three times—inductions, epidurals. They had been easy and gone well, but something was missing and this time she wanted it to be different. She wanted to try a waterbirth. Her pregnancy was uneventful except for the worst varicose veins I have ever seen, and I told myself that the water would be good for those. She showed up at the hospital at five in the morning, after I had had a long shift since the previous morning with four births, several of which had been difficult and disappointing. "Why did she have to go into labor now?" I asked myself.

She was clearly in active labor, and we filled the tub right away. I decided not to do a vaginal exam, but just to wait and see. She got in the tub with her husband. During the next two contractions, she said, "Oooh, this feels much better," but with the third she groaned and grunted, and I knew the baby was coming. "What about the amniotic fluid?" the nurse asked. We always rupture membranes before the baby comes to make sure there is not meconium in the fluid. "Look," I responded. "What do you think?" There was a huge, luminous, clear bubble with sparkling white flecks emerging from the woman's vagina under the water. The bubble continued to bulge out until we could see a head inside the bubble, stretching the perineum and slowly emerging into the water. For a few minutes, the baby stayed just like that, head inside the bubble under the water, eyes open and looking around, body still inside her mom. Then the woman pushed again as I swept the membranes away from the baby's face. As the body came out, we pulled this perfect baby girl up onto her mother's breast, head out of the water, body in. She never cried or squirmed, just continued to look around in wonder at the big new world she found herself in. She was pink from head to toe, fat, with just a little yellow fuzz on her round head.

I wish that all my births could be like that one. But I know that if they were, I would soon feel bored. I need the perfect births, but the ones that challenge me, that make me glad that I chose this path, are the difficult ones. I want to be with the women who would be alone if I were not there, or would not be treated with compassion and respect, or would be given unnecessary interventions, risky procedures. I want to be with the babies who would not be welcomed if I was not there to welcome them. Every woman deserves someone to be with her in childbirth; every baby deserves to be welcomed into this world. To be a midwife, to be the one who tries to fulfill these needs, is an enormous privilege, a great gift. I cannot imagine taking a different path.

CHOOSING A MIDWIFE: A PHYSICIAN'S PERSPECTIVE

by Regula E. Burki, MD, FACOG

Midwifes have delivered babies for thousands of years. Women would turn to the person in the group who had the most experience with child birth who then became the designated midwife and gained further experience as time went on. This experience would be passed on to an apprentice. In some indigenous cultures the tribe's "midwife" to this day is a man.

An interesting book on the early history of midwives is *Witches, Midwives, and Nurses: A History of Women Healers* by Barbara Ehrenreich and Deirdre English. The same authors also wrote *Complaints and Disorders: The Sexual Politics of Sickness* on the history of female health care. Both these books are short and rather inflammatory—a delightful read!

As humanity has learned more about medicine and how the body works in general, and pregnancy and childbirth in particular, delivering babies has become more specialized. As a result, neonatal mortality has dropped from three digit numbers per thousand to one digit numbers in those areas of the world with access to professionals trained and certified in pregnancy and childbirth and facilities that can mount a high-tech response when necessary. Where those services are not available, or not affordable, infant and maternal mortality and injury remain appallingly high.

For several decades in the twentieth century, the process of child birth became more and more medicalized by the U.S. medical profession. At the extreme, women gave birth so heavily drugged, that they were unable to push, had their babies dragged out of them with forceps and could (luckily?) hardly remember giving birth! The stereotype of the expectant father was a chain-smoking, pacing man, far removed from the birthing area. As the result of a consumer revolt and with the arrival of more women in the medical profession, the situation has greatly changed. Birth has once again become a natural event. We now have fathers fully involved in the birthing process, including being present during C-sections. Well-equipped, home-like birthing rooms are now the norm, while high-tech emergency technology is readily available, should it become necessary. With the development of spinal and epidural anesthesia, for those women who desire it, the use of sedation has greatly diminished—to the benefit of both mothers and babies and their ability to bond immediately after birth.

Unlike in decades past, when doctors considered natural childbirth backwards and dangerous, the overwhelming majority of physicians practicing obstetrics nowadays are very comfortable with and supportive of natural childbirth and can provide you with a birthing experience as natural as you want it. They can also get you an epidural anesthesia if "natural" turns out to be more than you bargained for and you change your mind.

The birthing specialists most devoted to natural childbirth are the midwives. The trend to more births being attended by midwives (from 1% of all births in 1975 to 8% in 2001 according to the National Center for Health Statistics) is part of the consumer revolt against the medicalization of childbirth that took place in the early 1970s.

While it is true that poor and uninsured women are more likely to use midwives to deliver their babies, the relationship between socio-economic status and the use of midwives may not be as straightforward as previously thought.

Caucasian women on Medicaid are three times more likely than those paying with private insurance to use a certified nurse-midwife (CNM). Non-white women on Medicaid are five times more likely to use a CNM. The effect of education on midwife use also varied by race: A college education significantly increased the likelihood of midwife use among white women, but higher education decreased that probability among non-white women.

Unfortunately, the training, certification, expertise and experience of the various types of midwives offering to deliver your baby are far from transparent. Also, who is allowed and/or licensed to deliver babies varies from state to state, as does whose services are covered by insurance carriers.

Here is some basic information about the training and certification of midwives. For more extensive research, I recommend the websites listed at the end of this section and their links.

CERTIFIED NURSE MIDWIFE (CNM)

Certified nurse-midwives are registered nurses who have graduated from a midwifery education program accredited by the ACNM Division of Accreditation and have passed a national certification examination administered by the ACNM Certification Council (ACC). All ACNM accredited midwifery training programs are university affiliated and many award master's level degrees. The American College of Nurse-Midwives is a highly respected professional organization whose origins go back to the 1920s and represents over 7,000 members.

CERTIFIED MIDWIFE (CM)

CMs are trained in the same accredited, university-affiliated midwifery programs as certified nurse midwives are, have completed the same national certification exam as CNMs and adhere to the same professional standards as certified nurse-midwives.

They differ from CNMs only in that they are not registered nurses, but have a different, usually also health-related, undergraduate degree. They must fulfill prerequisite health science requirements before being admitted into an ACNM accredited midwifery training program. They are a distinct category of direct-entry midwife, and the only DEMs eligible for membership in the American College of Nurse-Midwives. As CMs are a relatively new entity, they are not yet recognized by many insurance carriers and, therefore, their services are often not covered.

The great majority of CNMs/CMs delivers in hospitals and birthing centers. The American College of Nurse-Midwives does have a standing committee on home birth and does not discourage its members from participating in home births, but few CNMs/CMs do it. For more information on CNM/CMs providing home births, check the ACNM website listed below.

All CNMs/CMs have a collaborative agreement with one or more physicians that clearly defines consultation and referral criteria based on the individual needs of each patient. This has been the practice for decades and generally is a condition for CNM/CMs to gain hospital admission privileges.

In October 2002, the American College of Obstetricians and Gynecologists (ACOG) and the American College of Nurse-Midwives (ACNM) released a joint statement again stressing the importance of such collaborative arrangements.

Direct-Entry Midwife (DEM)

The term DEM is often used collectively for all midwifes who do not meet the educational and training criteria to take the national certification examination administered by the ACNM Certification Council (ACC) and become members of the American College of Nurse-Midwives.

They include lay midwives, Granny Midwives, Spiritual Midwives, Apprentice-Trained Midwives (ATMs), Wicca Midwives, Certified Professional Midwives (CPMs), Licensed Practical Midwives (LPMs), etc. The terms, legal status and conditions of licensure vary from state to state. There are significant variations in levels of education, training, experience and scope of practice, which potentially impact outcomes.

In 1987, the Midwives' Alliance of North America (MANA) and the Midwifery Education and Accreditation Council (MEAC) joined together to create an alterative direct-entry midwifery credentialing process, in an effort to identify standards and practices for the independent midwifery community. It created the North American Registry of Midwives (NARM), which awards the credential of Certified Professional Midwife (CPM). The NARM certification process recognizes multiple routes of entry into midwifery and includes verification of knowledge and skills and the successful completion of both a written examination and skills assessment. The CPM credential requires training in out-of-hospital settings. Many states now accept CPM certification as a condition for licensure.

A whole host of midwifery schools, colleges and other institutions have sprung up around the country to train DEMs. They are not university affiliated, have their own credentialing agency and vary greatly in the quality of education they provide. It is therefore important to be cautious when reading studies about midwifery outcome statistics. In Europe, where midwives have always been much more common than in the U.S., the training of midwives is generally at the level of CNM. Thus a European-trained midwife cannot be compared with an apprentice-trained midwife in the U.S. who delivers only a few babies a year.

Just do the math: According to the National Center for Health Statistics, in 2001, there were 4.025 million births in the U.S., with 322,075 (8%) of them delivered by midwives. Of the midwife deliveries, 95% were by 5,700 certified nurse midwives, leaving a total of 16,103 babies to be delivered by midwives other than CNM/CMs. With an estimated 3,000 so-called direct-entry midwives (DEMs) practicing in the U.S., that leaves an average of 5.3 deliveries a year by these types of midwives. With this being the average number, many lay and other types of DEMs must be delivering only one or two babies a year, hardly enough to keep up their skills. Compare this to an average of 53.6 per year for CNM/CMs and about double that amount for the average obstetrician.

DEMs are the main providers of home births. Many DEMs are limited in their practice sites, as they generally do not have hospital admission privileges and often have no collaborative arrangements with a physician. Few physicians are willing to provide back-up services for DEMs thus taking on the medical and legal risk of being the perceived "deep pocket" in a situation involving home birth and sometimes marginal training on the part of the DEM.

Nevertheless, many DEMs are highly experienced and provide valuable services to sectors of the community that have no access to other types of care, either because of socio-economic or immigration status or religious or cultural norms.

My personal recommendation is that if you want your baby delivered by a midwife, choose a certified nurse-midwife or a Certified Midwife, as did 95% of all women whose babies were delivered by a midwife in 2001. The training and certification process for CNMs and CMs is comparable in its intensity and rigor to the training of obstetrician/gynecologists. This is recognized by the fact that members of the American College of Nurse-Midwives are welcomed as educational affiliates of the American College of Obstetricians and Gynecologists.

The training and certification process of direct-entry midwives is much less clear and may vary greatly, as does their experience level.

In many states, lay midwives operate in a confusing legal situation, where they are allowed to deliver babies, but not to administer any prescription medications, though many administer prescription medication illegally. In Utah, for example, they tend to provide home births for a subculture on the fringe of society, including the polygamist community. Emergency on call doctors end up taking care of the severe complications that sometimes arise. Because of the ambiguous legal situation, the women usually arrive at the hospital far too late to save the situation and the outcomes tend to be disastrous. The doctors greatly resent being forced to deal with these desperate calamities, especially because often they end up being sued on top of the emotional strain of being too late to help! As a result of the legal risks involved, lay midwives, unlike certified nurse-midwives and certified midwives, rarely have cooperative agreements and backup arrangements with physicians, which puts their patients further at risk.

Useful websites for finding more information on training and certification of the different types of midwives include:

http://www.acnm.org: American College of Certified Nurse-Midwives home page. This is the organization that represents the certified nurse-midwives and the certified midwives. If you are interested in a home birth, follow their link to the ACNM homebirth committee. It provides a list of CNMs who provide home births.

http://www.accmidwife.org: American College of Certified Nurse-Midwives Certification Council (ACNM-ACC) home page. To learn more about the CNM/CM certification exam, click on Candidate Booklet, then Test Outline. This site also has information about the process required to maintain certification.

http://www.narm.org: North American Registry of Midwives home page. This is the organization that represents the direct-entry midwives (DEMs). This site also lists the educational requirements for becoming a certified professional midwife (CPM).

http://www.midwife.org/prof/display.cfm?id=208: The site defines commonly used acronyms, which is helpful in sorting out the alphabet soup of various birthing professionals and their organizations.

DOULAS

from Doulas of North America

WHAT IS A DOULA?

The word "doula" comes from ancient Greek and is now used to refer to a woman experienced in childbirth who provides continuous physical, emotional, and informational support to the mother before, during and just after childbirth. Studies have found that when doulas attend births, labors are shorter with fewer complications. There is less need for oxytocin to speed labor, forceps or vacuum extractor deliveries, pain medication or epidurals, and cesarean deliveries. Babies are healthier and they breast-feed more easily.

A Birth Doula

- Recognizes childbirth as a key experience the mother will remember all her life.

- Understands the physiology of birth and the emotional needs of a woman in labor.
- Assists the woman in preparing for and carrying out her plans for the birth.
- Stays with the woman throughout labor.
- Provides emotional support, physical comfort measures, and an objective viewpoint, as well as helping the woman get the information she needs to make informed decisions.
- Facilitates communication between the laboring woman, her partner and clinical care providers.
- Perceives her role as nurturing and protecting the woman's memory of the birth experience.

The acceptance of doulas in maternity care is growing rapidly with the recognition of their important contributions to the improved physical outcomes and emotional well-being of mothers and infants. They are found in many settings, from the home to the hospital, and work in cooperation with doctors, nurses, midwives, and the partners of laboring women.

Some doulas also provide postpartum care and support to a family with a newborn baby.

How to Find a Doula

For a referral to a doula in your area, contact Doulas of North America (DONA) at www.dona.org or the DONA Central Office at:

P.O. Box 626
Jasper, Indiana 47547
(888) 788-dona (3662), doula@dona.org

Doulas of North America is an international non-profit organization of doulas who are trained to provide the highest quality labor support to birthing women and their families. DONA was founded in 1992.

The main purposes of DONA are to certify doulas using an international standard; to facilitate continuing education; and to provide a strong communication link among practicing doulas, the childbearing public, maternity caregivers and others interested in learning about labor support. In these ways, DONA meets an important need in maternal health care by increasing the availability of trained doulas in North America and helping pregnant women find them.

QUESTIONS TO ASK A DOULA

The following questions will help you decide if a particular doula is right for you. You may choose to ask these questions over the phone before having an in-person interview.
- What training have you had?
- Tell me (us) about your experience with birth, personally and as a doula?
- What is your philosophy about childbirth and supporting women and their partners through labor?
- May we meet to discuss our birth plans and the role you will play in supporting me (us) through childbirth?
- May we call you with questions or concerns before and after the birth?
- When do you try to join women in labor? Do you come to our home or meet us at the hospital?
- Do you meet with me (us) after the birth to review the labor and answer questions?
- Do you work with one or more backup doulas (for times when you are not available)? May we meet her/them?
- What is your fee?

Your doula will be with you throughout labor and the birth of your baby. We encourage you to meet with your doula prenatally. Because she is helping to create the intimacy of your birth experience, it is particularly important that you and your partner feel comfortable with her personality. You may want to interview more than one doula in person.

DOULA STATISTICS

Benefits of having a trained doula:
50% reduction in the cesarean rate
25% shorter labor
60% reduction in epidural requests
40% reduction in oxytocin use
30% reduction in analgesia use
40% reduction in forceps delivery

From Mothering the Mother: How a Doula Can Help You Have a Shorter and Healthier Birth, Klaus, Kennell, and Klaus (1993).

A Doula's Tale: Mary

by Mary Paliescheskey, BS, BG

The phone rings in the middle of the night. What time is it? I answer it and try to drag myself from the blanket of sleep. It's my client. She awakened to some contractions. We talk for a while as I slowly awaken and answer her questions and concerns. Her questions revolve around "Is it time now?" and "How will I know?" We talk some more. The contractions seem to be mild, so I recommend she go back to sleep and we will talk again in the morning.

I hang up and look over at my husband. He didn't even flinch when the phone rang. Phone calls in the night just mean a client is due. He mumbles a question. I pat him and say, "no not yet."

As I breathe myself back to sleep, I think of all the families I have helped over the years. I have helped couples find their own ways to birth. I have helped them laugh their babies out, use hypnosis, water births, first-time moms, second- or more time-moms, VBACs, C-sections, no interventions, or many technologies needed. It is all so individual. I always find it hard to describe what I do. The thing that is the same is that they are all looking for security and confidence.

I call my client in the morning and find that it was Braxton Hicks [also known as "false labor"]. She is not in active labor. We talk, and I assure her that it is absolutely no problem to call me in the middle of the night. That's why I'm here.

We talk several times over the week. Then one evening, I get a call from her husband. He's not sure if it's labor this time, so many times the contractions went away. No question in my mind. My client wants to go to the hospital. I say I'll meet them there. This is it. My client was unable to talk on the phone. Her contractions were calling her attention.

Normally I go to my client's home and then move with them to the hospital, but this mom wants to get to the hospital now. I have learned in my years of practice that the mother always knows best. I grab my bag and leave the house.

During the labor, I help with positions, back support, conversation, shower, food, and hydration. We walk the halls. We talk about babies. We talk about hopes and dreams. We talk about fears and concerns. Yes we'd talked about these things before in the prenatal appointments. A lot of things are cleared up and concerns met at that time. Sometimes things surface in birth and become suddenly important.

I have learned that my vocation is not just about knowledge of birth and position changes. I am part best friend, part doula, part psychologist, part sister, and a dash of mother all mixed together. I provide unconditional support.

This birth goes smoothly and very fast. As usual, the mother is right. Her child is born a few hours after arriving, without medications or other complications. Most births end up being uncomplicated.

Mother and father greet the baby. Their faces glow with love, adoration, and pride. This is what it is all about—the moment that the family is created. I am honored to witness this beautiful event many times a year.

As I watch this family grow, I think about how women are vulnerable during their labors and how some of them have set goals and expectations. I have held women as they cried because they failed to meet their own expectations. They grieve that they felt the need for medication. They express a sense of failure at their need, and ask my permission to take medication. My permission. Who am I to withhold my permission? I hold the ones who need holding and nurture them through the process. It is their own permission that they are really asking for because, as a doula, I never judge the choices.

Then this mother turns to me and says, "I couldn't have done it without you." I reply with, "I'm glad my presence helped you." Inside, I smile and think that it wasn't me at all. I was simply the guide that allowed her to trust this process.

For more information contact:
Mary Paliescheskey, Birth Guide
Mothering the Mother Birth Services
617 15th St.
Huntington Beach, CA 92648
numbers@rocketmail.com, http://members.tripod.com/doula

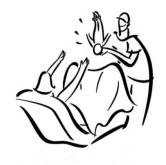

Part Three: Choices of Birth Techniques

Choices of Birth Techniques

WHERE TO BEGIN: CHILDBIRTH EDUCATION

Most people want to gather as much information as possible before the birth of their baby. Hospitals, various organizations and individuals provide a choice of classes that cover general health and nutrition, labor and delivery preparation, breast-feeding and newborn care.

ICEA

Some childbirth educators are certified by the International Childbirth Education Association (ICEA). This indicates that the person certified has achieved a certain level of knowledge and competency in areas tested by ICEA. ICEA certification does not indicate that the person certified is employed by ICEA. ICEA does not monitor, nor is it responsible for, the content of any classes, seminars or other presentations led or conducted by such persons or services provided by them.

ICEA's Goal and Philosophy

Family-centered maternity care is ICEA's primary goal and the basis of ICEA philosophy. In 1986, ICEA adopted the McMaster University definition of Family-Centered Maternity Care (FCMC).

Philosophy: The birth of a baby represents, as well, the birth of a family. The woman giving birth and the persons significant and close to her are forming a new relationship with new responsibilities to each other, to the baby, and to society as a whole. Family-centered reproductive care may be defined as care that recognizes the importance of these new relationships and responsibilities, and that has as its goal the best possible health outcome for all members of the family, both as individuals and as a group.

Family-centered care consists of an attitude, rather than a protocol. It recognizes a vital life event, rather than a medical procedure. It appreciates the importance of that event to the woman and to the persons who are important to her. It respects the woman's individuality and her sense of autonomy. It realizes that the decisions she may make are based on many influences, of which the expertise of the professional is only one. It requires that all relevant information be made available to the woman to help her achieve her own goals, and that she be guided, but not directed, by professionals she has chosen to share the responsibility for her care.

Practice: The practice of family-centered maternity care is founded on this philosophy and encompasses birth practitioners, birth places, and maternity-newborn care, as determined by the needs and choices of each woman and her family. Our goal is to support this type of family-centered care.

ICEA Mission Statement

The International Childbirth Education Association (ICEA) is a professional organization that supports educators and other health care providers who believe in freedom of choice based on knowledge of alternatives in family-centered maternity and newborn care.

ICEA's goals are to provide
- Professional certification programs
- Training and continuing education programs
- Quality educational resources

ICEA is a nonprofit, primarily volunteer organization. Since its formation in 1960, ICEA members and member groups have remained autonomous, establishing their own policies and creating their own programs. There are no membership requirements for individuals other than a commitment to family-centered maternity care and the philosophy of freedom of choice based on knowledge of alternatives in childbirth.

For a referral to a childbirth educator in your area, contact www.icea.org or phone (952) 854-8660.

Choosing Childbirth Education

To help you decide which childbirth class is for you, consider the comments below and select the top three areas you want a class to cover. Keep these in mind and they will help direct you to the most appropriate class for your needs.

- A hospital tour and introduction to what to expect once I arrive for the birth.
- Information about general health and nutrition during pregnancy.
- Information about the stages of labor and what to expect.
- Instruction in breathing and relaxation techniques.
- Discussion of different pain medications and options available.
- Discussion of natural childbirth.
- Discussion of water birth.

Birth Techniques

Discussed below are three well-known techniques that have been developed to help women through childbirth:

The Lamaze Method
The Bradley Method Husband-Coached Childbirth
Water Birth

Less known is hypnobirth, which is discussed at the end of this section. Which technique you choose may affect where you give birth. Water birth, for example, is not available in every hospital.

THE LAMAZE METHOD
from Lamaze International

The Lamaze Method was developed by Dr. Fernand Lamaze and combines learned breathing techniques with relaxation exercises designed to get a woman through labor comfortably.

LAMAZE INTERNATIONAL HISTORY & MISSION

Lamaze has changed childbirth for millions of families through the dedicated efforts of professional childbirth educators, providers and parents, since its founding as a nonprofit association in 1960. The birthing experience that we consider standard now—awake, aware, supported by family and friends, no maternal/infant separation—was unheard of in the United States when we began. Our cofounder and Emeritus Director, Elisabeth Bing, tells this pioneering story in her article *Lamaze Childbirth: Then and Now*.

The Lamaze mission is to promote normal, natural, healthy and fulfilling childbearing experiences for women and their families through education, advocacy and reform. Our mission is accomplished through:

Advocacy—Changing the birth culture by ensuring that the environment protects a woman's dignity and access to a full spectrum of comfort measures and continuous support.

Education—Enhancing the knowledge and skills of women, families and professionals through education and certification.

Reform—Transforming the birth culture by fostering those attitudes in society that enable families to have a positive birth, breast-feeding and parenting experience.

The work of the organization is carried out by Lamaze members and volunteer leaders—childbirth educators, nurses, nurse-midwives, physicians, students and consumers—who support Lamaze childbirth and parenting. One of the primary ways the organization pursues its mission is by training new childbirth educators through its internationally recognized Lamaze Childbirth Educator Program and Certification Examination. To date, Lamaze has educated and certified over 11,000 Lamaze Certified Childbirth Educators (LCCEs). The education program is currently offered through university and chapter programs throughout the United States, Canada and Mexico.

Lamaze has adopted philosophy statements on birth and parenting, which serve as the foundation for the work of the organization.

LAMAZE PARENTING PHILOSOPHY

- Good parenting is vital to the physical, emotional and spiritual health of our children, ourselves and our society.
- Parenting is joyful, important, challenging and deeply satisfying work that is worthy of everyone's best efforts.
- Parenting begins before birth. The intimate connection between children and their parents must be respected and protected from the moment of birth throughout life.
- Mothers and fathers play unique, irreplaceable roles in their children's lives.
- Babies and children thrive in close, consistent interaction with their parents.
- Parenting is a learned art; our most important teachers are our own parents, our family, and our children.
- Parenting requires the support of family, friends and community.
- Knowledge and support enhance parents' confidence and ability to make informed decisions that meet the needs of their children and themselves.

LAMAZE PHILOSOPHY OF BIRTH

- Birth is normal, natural and healthy.
- The experience of birth profoundly affects women and their families.
- Women's inner wisdom guides them through birth.

- Women's confidence and ability to give birth is either enhanced or diminished by the care provider and place of birth.
- Women have the right to give birth free from routine medical interventions.
- Birth can safely take place in birth centers and homes.
- Childbirth education empowers women to make informed choices in health care, to assume responsibility for their health and to trust their inner wisdom.

Lamaze Childbirth Class

If you are an expectant parent looking for a Lamaze childbirth education class, you can find a Lamaze Certified Childbirth Educator in your area at www.lamaze.org, our on-line locator service, by e-mailing the Lamaze Administrative Office at info@lamaze.org, or by calling us at (800) 368-4404.

Reprinted with the permission of Lamaze International.

5 Lamaze Myths
compiled by Lamaze International

There are five myths about Lamaze and the Lamaze birthing method that persist today. Here's the truth behind the myths.

Myth No. 1: Lamaze is all about breathing.
Myth No. 2: Lamaze promises painless childbirth.
Myth No. 3: Lamaze means you can't have an epidural.
Myth No. 4: Lamaze doesn't work.
Myth No. 5: Lamaze is not for everyone.

Myth No. 1: Lamaze is all about breathing.

Reality: The goal of Lamaze classes is to increase women's confidence in their ability to give birth. Lamaze classes help women discover the inner wisdom they already have for giving birth. Women learn simple coping strategies for labor, including focused breathing. But breathing techniques are just one of many things that help women in labor. Movement and positioning, labor support, massage, relaxation, hydrotherapy, and the use of heat and cold are some others.

MYTH NO. 2: LAMAZE PROMISES PAINLESS CHILDBIRTH.
Reality: Many women are afraid of the pain that is a normal part of childbirth. The pain of labor and birth, like other pain, protects us. Responding to the pain of contractions—by changing positions and moving, by massaging, by moaning—actually strengthens the contractions, helps the baby settle into the pelvis and move through the birth canal, and reduces pain perception. Some women find that experiencing and coping with the pain of labor and birth is similar to the hard work demanded by dancers and athletes. Lamaze classes help women understand the value of pain and learn how to respond to pain in ways that both facilitate labor and increase comfort.

MYTH NO. 3: LAMAZE MEANS YOU CAN'T HAVE AN EPIDURAL.
Reality: Lamaze classes provide information about natural pain relief options, as well as epidural anesthesia. Eliminating pain completely makes it difficult to respond to contractions in ways that facilitate labor and birth. Women who have epidural anesthesia are required to have IV fluids and continuous electronic fetal monitoring. They may be encouraged to stay in bed and may need medications to increase the strength of contractions. The ability to use many of the comfort techniques learned in Lamaze classes, such as changing positions, walking, and hydrotherapy, may be limited. Lamaze education will assist women in making personal decisions that are right for them.

MYTH NO. 4: LAMAZE DOESN'T WORK.
Reality: Lamaze that "works" has nothing to do with feeling pain, taking or avoiding medication, or developing complications that necessitate medical interventions. Lamaze teaches women that nature has designed birth simply and close to perfectly and that women already know how to give birth. Lamaze is working if women trust the natural process of birth, have confidence in their ability to give birth, have the freedom to work with their bodies as labor progresses, and are supported by health care providers, family and friends who wait patiently for nature to do its incredible work. Lamaze "works" if birth is allowed to work.

MYTH NO. 5: LAMAZE IS NOT FOR EVERYONE.
Reality: Women have always prepared for the birth of their babies. Until recent times, women learned about birth from their own

mothers and sisters. Birth took place at home with family rituals and traditions to help them feel confident in their ability to give birth. Women were surrounded by family and wise women who provided comfort and encouragement through labor and in the days and weeks after birth. Today, Lamaze childbirth classes provide the knowledge, skills, and support that help women give birth with confidence and joy, as they have done for centuries. Lamaze preparation is for everyone!

Information reprinted with the permission of Lamaze International Inc. For more information contact
www.lamaze.org
lamaze@dc.sba.com
(800) 368-4404

THE BRADLEY METHOD®

from American Academy of Husband-Coached Childbirth

The Bradley Method was developed by Dr. Robert A. Bradley who co-founded The American Academy of Husband-Coached Childbirth with Marjie and Jay Hathaway for the purpose of making childbirth education information available.

THE BRADLEY METHOD'S CHILDBIRTH GOALS

Your currently affiliated Bradley instructor wants you and your baby to have the best, safest, and most rewarding birth experience possible (a healthy mother and baby are our primary goals). For that reason, we endorse and teach the following ideals in class:

1. Natural childbirth.
2. Active participation of the husband as coach.
3. Excellent nutrition, the foundation of a healthy pregnancy.
4. Avoidance of drugs during pregnancy, birth, and breast-feeding unless absolutely necessary.
5. Training: "Early-bird" classes followed by weekly classes starting in the sixth month, continuing until birth.
6. Relaxation and natural breathing.
7. "Tuning-in" to your own body.
8. Immediate and continuous contact with your new baby.
9. Breast-feeding beginning at birth.
10. Consumerism and positive communications.

11. Parents taking responsibility for the safety of the birth place, procedures, attendants and emergency backup.
12. Parents prepared for unexpected situations, such as emergency childbirth and cesarean sections.

Educated parents have the responsibility to make these choices themselves. They also need to seek personnel who have natural childbirth experience and who will support their choices. This may take considerable effort and sometimes requires seeking special personnel or traveling great distances to achieve the safest possible birth.

The Bradley Method recommends that informed parents consider the many choices available. These decisions may affect their lives and the life of their unborn child. Differences of opinion exist even among "experts" and many doctors have become burned-out on patients who say they want natural childbirth, but do not put the effort and dedication into realistic training. Your enthusiasm is contagious and, when combined with preparation and dedication, it can lead to a wonderful birthing experience.

Your local Bradley Method instructor is an independent professional person or couple trained to help pregnant couples obtain the birth experience they desire. These instructors have received intensive training by the American Academy of Husband-Coached Childbirth in natural childbirth, labor coaching and normal variations. They are required to re-affiliate each year in order to continue teaching the Bradley Method. Ask to see your instructor's current certificate of affiliation.

For the protection of the public, the terms "The Bradley Method" and "Husband-Coached Childbirth" have been registered. Only teachers currently affiliated with the Academy may teach The Bradley Method.

The Standard Class Series Course Content:
Class 1. *Introduction to The Bradley Method*
Class 2. *Nutrition in Pregnancy*
Class 3. *Pregnancy*
Class 4. *The Coach's Role*
Class 5. *Introduction to First Stage Labor*
Class 6. *Introduction to Second Stage Labor*
Class 7. *Planning Your Birth*
Class 8. *Variations and Complications/Postpartum Preparation*
Class 9. *Advanced First Stage Techniques*
Class 10. *Advanced Second Stage Techniques*

Class 11. *Being a Great Coach/Are You Ready?*
Class 12. *Preparing for Your New Family*
For a referral to a childbirth educator in your area contact:

American Academy of Husband-Coached Childbirth®
Box 5224
Sherman Oaks
CA 91413-5224
1-800-4-A-BIRTH, 818-788-6662
www.bradleybirth.com

WATER BIRTH

WATER BIRTH: A 10 YEAR RETROSPECTIVE

by Barbara Harper, RN

The First International Conference on Waterbirths, held in London in April, left me with a calm and inner satisfaction that is difficult to express. I sat in the darkened auditorium, surrounded by more than 1,000 birth practitioners from 36 countries, listening to reports and statistics from nearly 9,000 waterbirths. And I wept. Gut-wrenching tears spilled down my face. I felt an emotional release, an exhausted escape, caused by the realization that I was not alone in telling the world about the wonder of water. And I was encouraged by the people who wanted me to be successful, and who respected and supported my chosen path. The support overwhelmed me. But this has not always been so.

I was introduced to waterbirth in 1983, when I was shown the book *Water Babies* by Erik Sidenblah. This book chronicled the life and work of Russian Igor Charcovsky, a gym teacher, boat builder, researcher and scientist. Although not a physician, Charcovsky experimented extensively with the use of warm water immersion during the process of human labor. He wanted to observe the effects of buoyancy on laboring women. Gradually, he began allowing women to birth in his warm water-filled tubs. His focus shifted to observing newborn behavior, and he recommended that infants be immediately placed back into an aquatic environment.

I wanted to learn more about the benefits and risks of warm water immersion for labor and birth, so I traveled to Paris in search of Dr. Michel Odent and Dr. Frederick Leboyer, both familiar with labor and birth in water. I was unable to meet them, but I did talk with midwives who worked with Dr. Odent and with several mothers who had given birth in water. I also witnessed labor in water and nonmedical births.

My whole life changed on October 27, 1984, when I gave birth to my second child in a homemade water tub. I made a conscious decision to educate the public and medical professionals in this country, if not the world, on the efficacy and safety of birthing babies in warm water. This path was fraught with controversy, rejection and ridicule from both the medical establishment and the midwifery community.

Between 1984 and 1988, fifteen women came to my home to birth their babies in my hot tub. Hundreds more called and asked for help. I began teaching workshops and holding information nights in my home. Every woman who had a waterbirth influenced at least ten others to be curious about it. Then came Michel Odent's revolutionary book, *Birth Reborn*, at the end of 1984. Women finally had a model on which to base their instinctive desires for a completely natural birth experience in or out of the water.

In 1988, I went on my first trip to Russia to meet with parents who had had waterbirths. I also wanted to meet Igor Charcovsky. I met with dozens of parents and had a lengthy meeting with Igor. Midwives and parents took me to local hospitals, where I saw the incredible need for alternatives to the horrors of Soviet maternity care. During my trip, I also went to Crimea, where I was told many women gave birth in the Black Sea during the summer months. I saw no births during my brief visit, but I met more people in the waterbirth movement in Russia.

During that trip, I promised the Russian waterbirth couples and their midwives that I would found an international organization that might be able to help them gain recognition as a legitimate group by their own government. At the same time, I knew we needed a similar vehicle in the United States to disseminate correct and current information about labor and birth in water. When a negative commentary on waterbirth appeared in the Fall 1988 issue of *Mothering*, I responded with a compassionate letter sharing my personal experience and asking for interested people to contact me with stories of their own births or questions and comments. The positive mail I received was overwhelming and was the impetus for me to begin my nonprofit organization, Waterbirth International. Our intent was to preserve and protect natural childbirth and natural childbirth in water. To achieve that end, we would engage in charitable, educational, research and publishing activities.

Three years ago, we changed the name to the Global Maternal/Child Health Association (GMCHA) to more accurately reflect all that we do. Birth in water is simply a platform from which to inform a basically misinformed public on all the issues that surround birth. The public has become so used to seeing images on television of women being drugged, plugged, probed, prodded, managed and coached! But when someone sees a waterbirth on television, what he or she truly remembers is a woman empowered to reach down and lift up her own baby. The woman is awake and aware, she moves however she wishes, and has her chosen birth attendants supporting and watching her.

The whole picture of birth suddenly changed for thousands of women across America in 1993, when GMCHA helped produce a waterbirth segment for ABC's television show *20/20*.

Today, our focus is still the dissemination of current and correct information, but on a broader scale. The production of the video *Gentle Birth Choices* was a priority for us because it succinctly gave midwives the visual images and voices of authority and strength to help inform the public about the benefits of midwifery and natural childbirth. In addition, we provide a complete waterbirth information service and have been offering waterbirth courses and certification for midwives, nurses and doctors in and out of hospital settings. As more and more couples ask for warm water immersion, it is important to develop similar guidelines for practice, as well as for the installation and use of permanent tubs in hospital or clinic environments. Teaching remains very important, because technocracy won't change simply because tubs are installed. The rationales and research behind the reasons for allowing women to choose this option must be discussed.

To date, more than 250 midwives, 10 birth centers and 30 hospitals are listed on our U.S. referral list of practitioners who will help facilitate a waterbirth. ...

We are also creating a grant proposal that, if funded, would allow us to survey by mail and phone all the maternity units in the United States and Canada on the use of warm water as a pain management modality. Then we can start the painstaking process of tracking, using computer epidemiology programs, all waterbirths in all facilities, so that in the very near future we can have some usable retrospective data to offer the medical establishment. This has already been done in England through the National Perinatal Epidemiology Unit, a study funded by the British National Health Service. A true prospective randomized control trial of birth in water could be carried out on a very limited population; the model for that program has already been created in a small rural hospital in North Carolina. Within the next 25 years, it is our intent to see waterbirth become commonplace both in home birth and in clinical settings and to have several common "problems" in labor be an indication for a waterbirth.

One of my greatest pleasures has been my ability to meet the growing need for information as more and more women ask for waterbirths. Current global estimates on the number of waterbirths that have taken place in the last 10 years has grown as we discover low-key obstetricians and midwives around the planet who love using water for labor and birth. We now believe approximately 25,000 babies have been born in water between 1984 and 1995.

In early July, two Virginia traditional midwives attended the home birth of term twins, both born in water with breech presentations. One of the midwives said to me, as many midwives often say, "The more waterbirths I see in my practice, the less I want to do 'dry' birth." Gloria Lemay and Mary Sullivan, traditional midwives from Vancouver, British Columbia, followed the usual pattern of investigating waterbirth and becoming completely convinced of its relaxation, pain reduction and spiritual benefits. Almost all of their clients now request waterbirths; thus Gloria and Mary have attended close to 300 births in water.

Midwives who have not embraced waterbirth, or who choose not to allow women to stay in the tub for their births, have various personal and professional reasons. Midwives have challenged me at the start of my professional workshops with statements like, "I came here to decide if I am or am not going to do waterbirths. I'll let you know at the end of the workshop." I am not convincing anyone of anything. Rather, I am simply relating the information and letting people decide based on experience and comfort level. When teaching a waterbirth workshop, I begin with these remarks, "I want to tell you three things that waterbirth is not. It is not a fad—it is here to stay. It is not part of a cult—there is never just one way or a best way to give birth, for you or your baby. Waterbirth is not for everyone—mothers and practitioners alike."

Personally, I believe statistics don't matter; the medical establishment doesn't matter; the doubts and fears of others don't matter. What does matter is the innate wisdom women exhibit when given the opportunity to rid themselves of past or societal conditioning that inhibits and disempowers them. What does matter is the beauty of women giving birth in dignity, love and power, whether in or out of the water. And what matters is the manner in which babies are received.

I encourage women by telling them, "If water is your choice, your way, don't let someone else's attitude, fear or conditioning be an intervention to keep you from doing what is natural and normal for you." Our motto at Global Maternal/Child Health Association is, "Together, we're making a difference." It stands true for all of us concerned with keeping natural childbirth and waterbirth an option for our grandchildren and generations to come.

A Midwife's Perspective: Labor and Birth in the Water

by Jill Cohen

The benefits of water

It was late in the evening. I sat staring into the fire, waiting as I often do for the phone to ring. Midwives frequently have a sixth sense about birth, and on this particular evening, my senses proved true —at 10:30 p.m., the phone indeed rang. At first, all I heard was the echo of deep breaths and water running. I knew this was labor. Water and labor fit hand in hand for most laboring women. The shower or bath warms, secludes and relaxes a woman so she can open more easily at her own pace. It creates a womb-like environment in which a woman can feel safe. It may not take the pain away, but it enables a woman to cope through her intense sensations, relaxed and with least resistance, creating more comfort. Water forms a warm, wet buffer around her, keeping outside forces and interventions at bay. Yet if the woman should need assistance or monitoring, it can be accomplished easily in her watery environment.

I waited for the contraction to pass as I listened intently for the mystery woman on the other end of the phone to finally identify herself. I could tell by the echo that she was in her bathroom and could tell by the sound of running water that she was in the bath. The tempo of her breath told me I would be heading over soon ... as soon as I could ascertain who she was! After her breathing slowed and she paused to collect herself, I heard her giggle a "Sorry!" I knew right away it was my dear friend, Hazel. This was her fourth child—I was out the door!

Laboring in the water

I walked in to find her children sound asleep and her partner sitting at the edge of their large tub, a glass of cold water and bendable straw in hand to help keep Hazel well hydrated. Before she could utter a word, another contraction arrived and she went deep into herself. Because water can speed labor along once the woman is over five centimeters dilated, and I guessed that Hazel was at least that, I busied myself preparing her birthing room. I then settled into the bathroom with my water Doppler and monitored our little friend. All was well. Hazel needed to pee, so she got out and onto the toilet. Another big contraction, wide eyes and pop went the bag of waters. They were clear and smelled sweetly of baby. It was time to decide where this child would be born.

Without hesitation, Hazel chose the tub. As soon as she was situated, I heard the familiar sound of relief I hear so often when women sink into warm water. It is music to a midwife's ears, as is the steady heart rate of a baby about to be born. Hazel pushed with the next contraction as she pulled her legs back and sang that magical birth song, low and deep. With that push, we saw the baby's head. Two more pushes and the head was born.

As we waited for the next contraction, we had time to see this little child and appreciate the peacefulness of his or her entrance. Water is vital to life—we cannot live without it. Its ability to nourish, nurture, propagate and promote life fits so well in the birthing world. I believe that because babies come from a watery environment, when they are born into water it feels familiar to them. Under normal circumstances, babies will not breathe until they hit air. When they emerge into water, their house gets bigger, but they still think they are in the womb. This little one was wide-eyed and waiting. It is always amazing to see such peaceful passage.

Within a few moments, another contraction came and the baby was gently born. Hazel instinctively reached down and brought her baby to the surface. There was no need to suction—this little boy flexed, stretched, yawned and pinked up without even crying.

Misperceptions

Misunderstandings abound about the use of water in birth, such as risk of infection, risk to the baby, and lack of ability to monitor effectively. There is now much research-based evidence to indicate that, with proper preparation and protocol the risks are no more than for air birth. So for those women and practitioners who choose water to facilitate birth, go for it! But first, be informed: Investigate what standards should be used. Plan what kind of tub you will use, where to put it, and find your water source. Remember that water is a different medium to work with. Familiarize yourself with it; think about its potentials; imagine its relation to birth. Merge with it and feel its effects.

For me, the rewards of using water in labor and birth are summed up in that magic sound of relief in a woman's moan as she enters the warm water, and the magic moment as the baby comes forth with that peaceful look that tells me the passage has been safe and gentle.

Jill Cohen lives and practices midwifery in the Eugene, Oregon area. She is senior editor of The Birthkit *and associate editor of* Midwifery Today, *where this commentary originally appeared.*

For more information on water birth, see What I Learned From the First Hospital Birthing Pool *by Michel Odent, MD and* A Landmark in the History of Birthing Pools *by Michel Odent, MD.*

A Physician's Perspective on Water Birth

by Regula Burki, OB/GYN, FACOG

Anybody who has ever had sore muscles knows that a hot shower or bath is highly soothing. The muscle exertion of labor required in giving birth is no exception. Laboring women find hot showers and baths very helpful in easing their labor pain. Numerous publications, both lay and professional, report shorter labors and greater comfort when women are laboring immersed in water.

Nobody doubts that being born under water is appropriate for such marine mammals as whales and dolphins. Whether it is the best way for human babies to be born remains controversial.

The two points of concern are infection and water getting into the lungs of the baby born under water.

At this time, there are no randomized prospective studies comparing the outcomes of "land" versus "water" births. The published studies in the scientific literature are generally either compilations of positive experiences by advocates of water births or case reports of complications.

Web sites that advocate water birth have extensive, but not necessarily scientifically sound, explanations of how babies will not try to take their first breath while still under water. Nevertheless, there are several reports of near drownings and even some deaths in the medical literature. It appears that part of the problem is sometimes a delay in lifting the baby out of the water. As soon as the placenta is separating from the uterine wall, which can take place minutes after birth, the baby no longer receives oxygen through the mother's blood. Even dolphin moms push their babies to the surface.

Advocates of water birth also tend to treat the problem of hygiene rather cavalierly. But birth is a messy process involving blood, amniotic fluid, urine and even the release of feces by the laboring woman. To clean the birthing tubs or pools between laboring women according to current OSHA (Occupational Safety and Health Administration) standards is a nearly impossible process and there are several reports of infections associated with contaminated birthing tubs.

Neither the American College of Obstetricians and Gynecologists nor the American College of Nurse-Midwives nor the American Academy of Pediatrics endorses the practice of water births at this time.

HYPNOBIRTH
HYPNOBIRTHING: WHAT IS IT AND HOW DOES IT WORK?

by Kerry Tuschhoff, HBCE

Mention labor and delivery to an expectant mom in her last trimester, and chances are good that her heart will begin to race, her mind to flood with concern and in some cases, panic. She knows that the day is coming when a force much bigger than herself will take over and her body will govern itself completely. For some women, this is a very fearful event; but for Hypnobirthing mothers, it is merely a challenge faced with confidence and trust.

Hypnobirthing is a childbirth method that uses hypnosis to eliminate pain and fear from the birthing experience. In the past, the word "hypnosis" conjured up images of stage hypnotists re-creating Elvis or mesmerizing others into embarrassing situations. Now it is common for hypnosis to be used therapeutically in many areas of medicine, dental anesthesia and personal therapy sessions. Even so, there are many misconceptions regarding hypnosis that can dissuade those contemplating this powerful tool. Here are a few facts:

- All hypnosis is self-hypnosis; the hypnotherapist is only the guide. A person chooses to enter into a hypnotic state, stay in and come out at will.
- Approximately 90-95% of the population can be hypnotized. Willingness, belief and motivation have great influence over hypnotizability.
- During hypnosis you are neither asleep nor unconscious and will always "come out" when you wish.
- Stronger-minded and stronger-willed people are easier to hypnotize, not the other way around as is usually assumed.
- You cannot be made to divulge information or do anything against your will while in hypnosis.
- Hypnosis is not Satanic or religion oriented at all.

What is HypnoBirthing?

Hypnobirthing teaches an understanding of how the birthing muscles work in perfect harmony, as they were designed to do, when the body is sufficiently relaxed. The depth of relaxation necessary can easily be achieved with hypnosis, so couples learn these skills in classes and practice them at home every day until the baby arrives. The Birth Companions, as the partners are called, have a very integral role in the preparation process: listening to the audio tapes, reading the hypnobirthing book and handouts and guiding the mother into hypnosis with hypnosis scripts. They are also an invaluable part of the labor and birthing process, as they help the mother to focus and concentrate, as well as support her physically. All aspects of labor and birth are covered in class, as well as information on nutrition, exercise, avoiding complications, fear release sessions, birth plans and consumer issues.

Fear and expectation

In other cultures, childbirth is regarded as a natural, normal event in a woman's life. Birthing women are given support from other women, and children are often present to witness the event. In this way, birth is celebrated and honored. Young girls then grow up with the belief system that birth is a positive event in a woman's life, and their expectations of childbirth reflect this attitude. As a result, their births are similar to their predecessors—without pain and fear. They have a positive expectation of childbirth. In our culture, it is very much the opposite. For many generations, we have been told that delivering a baby is many hours of painfully agonizing work to be faced with fear and trepidation. We have heard stories from well-meaning friends and family that send shivers up our spines; and so the legacy continues. We experience pain in childbirth in part because we very much expect to!

In hypnobirthing, the expectant couple is taught to surround themselves with only positive people and messages to create a positive view of childbirth and the expectation that their birthing will be the beautiful, peaceful experience that nature intended. Our Fear Release Sessions are integral to this process, as they allow each person to address fears they have, work through possible solutions and then release them. Fear in labor can create tension, which creates pain, then more fear, and the cycle continues. Fear and anxiety can also create adrenaline production in the body, causing the labor to become dysfunctional, a common reason for cesarean section surgery. Freedom from fear can make a huge difference in the birthing experience.

Women are taught how to bring themselves into self-hypnosis instantly and create their own natural anesthesia whenever and wherever they need it. This is important, as any drugs taken by a laboring woman can be dangerous for her, and especially her baby. She has total control over her body and is an active participant in her birth process. As labor progresses, she goes deeper inside herself, trusting in her body's natural ability to give birth with ease and comfort. Her mind is programmed to give her exactly what she needs.

Too good to be true?

Can women give birth without experiencing pain? They can, but there are many variables in labor and birth that can affect the outcome, and couples need to have a positive but realistic view of hypnobirthing. Without a doubt, all mothers using hypnosis are much calmer and more relaxed during labor, which automatically creates more comfort, as well as having powerful post-hypnotic suggestions to actually eliminate pain and fear. How effective is this? Statistics vary for each class depending on the length of classes and the skill of the hypnobirthing Practitioner (as well as the dedication and compliance to the program of each birthing couple). Instructors can have backgrounds in hypnotherapy, nursing, message therapy, labor assistance or childbirth education. They are all then trained in hypnosis for childbirth and become Certified HypnoBirthing Practitioners. Not all women can have a pain-free birth, but most can have an easier, faster and much more comfortable one, especially important to those choosing home birth with a midwife.

Benefits of hypnobirthing

- Fewer drugs or no drugs at all means less risk of side effects on mother and baby.
- Shorter labors—resistance of the birthing muscles as a response to pain is minimized.
- An awake, energized mother due to total relaxation.
- A calm, peaceful birthing environment.
- Breech and posterior babies can be turned using hypnosis.
- Fewer interventions and complications during labor.
- Babies who are better sleepers and nursers due to fewer drugs in their systems.

It is well worth the time to research hypnosis as an option for labor. It is important to remember that all drugs given to a woman in labor reach the baby in less than five minutes in an adult dose, so using HypnoBirthing techniques can help avoid them. HypnoBirthing relaxation has even helped many a nervous dad to cope, as they experience hypnosis in class as well! In addition, the skills learned for relaxation and hypnosis can benefit new mothers with recovery and breast-feeding, and can be used in many everyday situations.

Kerry Tuschhoff has taught natural childbirth for more than 11 years and is Operations Director of Hypnobabies Network in Stanton, CA. (714) 898-2229.

www.hypnobabies.com, hypnobabies@attbi.com.
Information reprinted with permission of Kerry Tuschhoff.

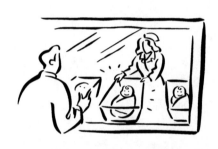

Part Four: Choices of Where to Give Birth

Choices of Where to Give Birth

by Barbara Harper, RN

Today, more women are successfully negotiating for the kind of birth experience they want. One choice is to have your baby at a hospital. Other choices include having your baby at a birthing center or at home.

HOSPITALS

In the last decade, many couples have succeeded in having satisfying birth experiences within an institutional setting. More and more hospitals are remodeling their birthing units. They are providing rooms in which the mother may labor, give birth and stay with her baby after birth.

Some of these birthing units, however, have become masterful reproductions of homelike environments that merely conceal the standard hospital technology. Everything needed for a medically controlled birth either pops out of the wall or conveniently rolls into the room. You must be aware of whether a hospital just advertises the availability of a gentle birth or truly provides it.

Make sure you talk with both the hospital and your doctor, so that you feel confident that you will be allowed to create the experience you want within the hospital. Some doctors will sit with women in labor and let the process unfold in an undisturbed way. Many hospitals also employ certified nurse midwives in their clinics.

Don't be dependent on your doctor to tell you everything about the hospital. Call the administration yourself and ask about the hospital's policies and whether tours of the maternity area are offered. Even if you have a great relationship with your doctor and you write a detailed birth plan, you may be faced with the limits of hospital policy the minute you are admitted. You might set aside some time to visit the maternity unit and talk to some of the nurses who work there. Talk to other women who have given birth at that hospital.

When you talk with anyone affiliated with the hospital, write down your questions so you know what to ask. By asking questions, sometimes simple ones, you make the hospital staff more aware of the growing concerns for gentle birth choices.

BIRTHING CENTERS

There is great client satisfaction at birthing centers. The homelike atmosphere and relaxed attitudes help make women feel safe. Women bring their personal items, chosen music, and, most importantly, any and all of their family members.

The following description of a freestanding birth center in California is typical of what you will find at the many birth centers now available across the country:

A sunny patio with a tiled fountain greets visitors and clients as they enter the birthing center. A tour of the center conducted by the center's founder, a board-certified obstetrician and gynecologist, reveals a warmly decorated interior, including three large birthing rooms with double beds and private toilets and showers. There are two separate bathrooms, each with large fiberglass bathtubs. The large classroom is full of very pregnant women and their partners watching a film on birth.

The kitchen is abundantly stocked with juices, fruit, cookies and other snacks, and the waiting area is filled with comfortable couches and chairs. The nerve center of this facility is located behind three walls of glass, where the telephone and the busy staff can be faintly heard. Everything is immaculately clean and fresh, with colors that are harmonious, warm and restful. Large color photographs of mothers, fathers and newborn babies decorate the walls. They were taken by the founder.

In the reception area, an older man and woman were anxiously waiting to enter one of the birthing rooms. Their daughter, who happened to be a pediatrician, had just given birth to their second grandchild. The sounds of a newborn and the happy murmuring of his loving family could be clearly heard. On another couch in the reception area, a man and woman were holding a tiny, peaceful baby who had been born at the center just the day before.

The founder worked hard in the beginning to convince women that they have the ability to birth their babies without technology and drugs. Many of the women were afraid that they would not be able to give birth without an epidural for pain. At first, women were given the option of childbirth education classes at the birthing center. After a few years, the founder noticed that the women who actively participated in the classes, especially for their first pregnancies, had much easier births than those women who just came for their regularly scheduled prenatal visits. He now insists that all women participate in prenatal education.

The founder sees the classes at the birthing center as more than teaching women how to give birth—they reinforce the normalcy of birth. The classes provide an experience of support that allows couples to feel comfortable in the birthing environment. Pregnant women often stop by the center to discuss some of their concerns about their anticipated births over a cup of tea. The importance of a casual relationship to the birthplace and the care providers cannot be underestimated. Each time a mother drops by or has a prenatal visit, the birthing center becomes more familiar. When she eventually arrives to have her baby, she does not have to cope with adjusting to a strange place.

During a prenatal class, a birth will often be taking place down the hall. If a woman calls in early labor, the phone call is answered by the founder personally. You can hear him telling her to be sure to eat, to rest if she is tired, and to call back when the contractions are longer, more intense and closer together. He finishes by saying, "I'll probably see you tonight."

When the laboring woman arrives at the center, she and her partner and any other companions are taken to a birthing room. She is allowed to wear her own clothes and can decorate the room with personal possessions. She is also encouraged to eat lightly, and fluids are made readily available. Women may move freely during all stages of labor and can give birth in whatever position they choose. Infants are not separated from their mothers after the birth except for valid medical reasons. One of the only "rules" that is actively enforced at the birthing center is the requirement that the mother and baby stay for a full six hours after the birth. If complications are going to develop with the baby, they will usually occur within the first few hours.

The founder and others feel that birthing centers such as these will play a big part in the future of gentle birth.

Home Births

Why have a home birth?

Women who want to be in charge of every element in their environment often elect to have their babies at home. Many couples find that their desire for privacy and intimacy is the most important factor in their decision.

Is home birth legal?

Home birth is absolutely legal. The legal gray area depends on the status of midwives in each state. The midwife who provides prenatal care and attends the home birth assumes the legal responsibility for the life of the mother and baby. If there is no midwife involved, the parents then become legally responsible if anything happens to the baby during the birth.

Who will provide medical backup?

Some couples who are committed to home birth hire a midwife, but also see an obstetrician throughout their pregnancy just so they have help available in case of an emergency. When midwives work independently, without doctor help, they must rely on the doctors in the local emergency room to take over if there is a complication that requires transport to a hospital. A midwife who develops a working relationship with a doctor and hospital is considered a respected member of the healthcare team. Her presence and expertise are not only acknowledged but called upon.

What supplies are necessary?

Not much is really needed. Home birth kits are readily available from birthing supply companies. The kits contain:

- sterile gloves
- gauze pads
- a cotton hat for the baby
- drop cloths
- waterproof covers for the bed
- a thermometer
- a pan for sitz baths after birth

Midwives bring everything else needed, including the technology of birth, to the home. Fetal heart tones are monitored with fetoscopes or ultrasonic stethoscopes. Oxygen tanks stand ready in case either mother or baby needs oxygen. Midwives carry drugs that can be administered to slow or stop a hemorrhage. Most midwives also bring with them special herbal preparations, homeopathic remedies, massage techniques and even acupuncture needles. IV lines can be started at home; tears or episiotomies can be stitched.

Choosing to have a home birth demands commitment, cooperation and trust. For many couples, it is the most satisfactory choice. Many couples who have one or two births in the hospital and then try a home birth come away with a confidence that is unparalleled.

Reprinted with permission of Barbara Harper, RN.

ACOG'S POSITION ON HOME BIRTHS

The risk of death to newborns delivered at home is nearly twice that of newborns delivered in hospitals, according to a study in the August issue of *Obstetrics & Gynecology*. Newborns delivered at home were also at higher risk for having low Apgar scores—an assessment of the newborn's heart rate, breathing, muscle tone, reflexes and skin color within minutes of being born.

Researchers studied birth data from Washington State for the period 1989 to 1996. They compared outcomes of 7,518 infants intended to be born at home to the outcomes of 14,038 infants intended to be born in the hospital. They found that pregnant women intending to deliver at home were, on average, more likely to be married, white, nonsmokers, and to have other children.

Infants intended to be born at home were at higher risk for very low Apgar scores, a potentially fatal problem. The association between newborn death and intent to deliver at home was particularly strong for women with no previous births (nulliparous). Women were more likely to themselves experience problems, including prolonged labor and postpartum hemorrhage. According to the researchers, their study suggests that planned home births are associated with a higher risk of negative outcomes for both women and newborns.

Contact: Jenny Pang, MD, MPH, Department of Epidemiology, Washington School of Public Health, Seattle, WA, at jwpang@u.washington.edu.

—American College of Obstetrics and Gynecology News Release, 7/21/02

An OB's Perspective: Why I Would Have My Baby ONLY at a Hospital

by Regula Burki, MD, FACOG

I am a board-certified obstetrician/gynecologist, and I would never even consider a home birth for any of my patients or for myself. I had all of my three children in a well-equipped hospital birthing room with my husband holding my hand and hospital housekeeping cleaning up the mess afterwards. I did not have to buy a new mattress, nor a new carpet in my bedroom.

With the first child, I stayed three days, first, because managed care still allowed a three day stay back then, and second, because the nurses enjoyed teaching their OB/GYN intern what to do with her own baby! The intern was grateful, as I had never changed a diaper up to the birth of my first child. With the third child, I left the next morning. The insurance was pleased.

With all three of my children, I picked a hospital that had a neonatal nursery with a newborn specialist physician (neonatologist) in house. The great majority of babies can deliver themselves, but the ones that need help need it *now* and may need a lot of it. My second baby was intubated within minutes of his birth because he had a rare problem unique to newborn babies and would not breathe well on his own. Twenty-four hours later, the breathing tube was removed and he started nursing. A day later, we both went home. Now he is a national merit scholar. Had he been born at home, the means of giving his brain the oxygen it needed when he needed it would not have been available.

I feel strongly that parents have no right to put their children's brains at risk for the sake of having a "birthing experience at home," when safer, and perfectly acceptable, alternatives are now available. When I hear upper-class suburbia obsess about birthing procedures, I am reminded of my days as a resident at Harvard: The working class women came to the hospital to have a healthy baby; the yuppies came with a birthing plan focusing on their own birthing experiences. More often than not, giving birth was their first introduction to the fact that life with a baby rarely goes as planned!

Thanks to consumer pressure, the days are long gone when, drugged out of their minds, women had their babies dragged out of them by forceps because they were too out of it to push. A woman can have a home birth-like experience in a beautiful hospital or birthing center birthing room that is likely much nicer than her own bedroom! She can walk around, use a birthing chair or lie in bed with an epidural. She can get a massage or take a hot shower. She can have her loved ones present to support her, including her birthing coach. She can make home movies and look at herself giving birth in an overhead mirror. Her baby can be delivered by a certified midwife or a doctor, and her partner can help guide the baby out of her and cut the cord. But if there is a problem, discreetly hidden emergency equipment is right there and emergency personnel are next door. Problems can happen and they can happen fast. A uterus can rupture, a placenta can separate from the wall of the uterus, and the mom can have a pulmonary embolus or a seizure. Minutes can make the difference between normal life, death or brain damage.

The life expectancy of women in the U.S. is now almost twice as long as it was a hundred years ago. Much of this change can be attributed to a drastic decrease of death from childbirth. Pregnancy- and childbirth-related deaths are still the major producers of orphans in the developing world, where birth in a well-equipped hospital with trained professionals assisting is rarely available.

In 1950 in the U.S., 32.5 per 1,000 newborns died during birth or within the first week after birth (perinatal mortality). Now that number is 6.2 for whites and 13.1 for blacks. These are overall numbers and do not separate high- and low-risk births.

The perinatal mortality for low-risk births in the U.S. is now about 2.5-3 per 1,000. The internet is full of websites that claim that home birth is as safe as hospital birth. That may certainly be the case for some truly low-risk births in the hands of well-trained and experienced birth attendants. There are, however, other studies that show an increased risk, generally doubling, of neonatal death with home birth.

A persistent problem that shows up in many well-designed studies is the underestimation of risk. In an Australian study published in 1998, the perinatal death rate for home births was 7.1 per 1,000. The authors concluded that the main contributing factors to this high death rate were underestimation of risk associated with overdue babies, twins and breech position, and a lack of response to fetal distress. More than half of the babies in this Australian study died from asphyxia.

A study from Washington State published in 2002 found that low-risk babies born at home were twice as likely to die as babies born in the hospital (3.3 vs 1.7 per thousand). The babies born at home were also at higher risk for having low Apgar scores and their moms were at an increased risk for prolonged labor and hemorrhage. This study is particularly interesting because it excluded babies born at home by accident and only included babies that were deemed to be low-risk and were born at home intentionally. Those babies were compared to low-risk babies that were intentionally born in a hospital. It excluded twins and premies of less than 34 weeks. It also only included births that had a professional birth attendant, such as a midwife, nurse or physician. A frequent factor that is linked to the bad outcomes of home births is inexperienced lay attendants who only deliver a few babies a year.

The overwhelming majority of U.S. women have their babies in the safe, but now much more pleasant, environment of a hospital birthing room. According to the National Center for Health Statistics, 99 percent of births in 1997 were in hospitals, basically unchanged from 1989, but the percent of out-of-hospital births that took place at home increased, while those in freestanding birthing centers declined.

A freestanding birthing center can never provide the emergency intensive care that sometimes becomes necessary at a frightening speed. With the hospitals now offering birthing rooms as comfortable and luxurious as the freestanding centers, birth at a birthing center, with the inherent risk of transfer to a hospital by ambulance should things not go as smoothly as anticipated, becomes less attractive.

According to the National Hospital Discharge Survey, new moms are also beginning to stay in the hospital longer; after decreasing from 3.8 days in 1980 to 2.1 days in 1995, the average length of a hospital stay for childbirth increased to 2.4 days in 1997. After questions were raised about whether short stays, especially stays of one day or less, were endangering the health of mothers and babies, federal legislation was enacted in 1996 that prohibited insurers from restricting hospital stays for mothers and newborn infants to less than two days for vaginal deliveries or four days for cesarean deliveries.

The National Center for Health Statistics reports that while the vast majority of births in 2001 (91.3%) were attended by physicians, this proportion has declined steadily as the percent of births attended by midwives has slowly increased to account for 7.8% percent of all births in 2001. This number has steadily grown from 1% of all births in 1975. Ninety-five percent of midwife-attended births were by certified nurse-midwives. This percentage has remained stable over many years. For physician-attended births, the number attended by MDs has been dropping steadily, while those attended by DOs has been consistently increasing to 4.5% in 2000. Ninety-nine percent of all births in 2002 took place in a hospital. Of the 1% of out-of-hospital births, 29% percent were in freestanding birthing centers, 63% in residences, and the remainder presumably in transit.

The fact that more women choose to have their babies delivered by midwives reflects the trend to make childbirth a more personal and less "medical" procedure. I think this is wonderful, mostly because women now have a choice! A certified nurse midwife generally has a bachelor degree in nursing, followed by a graduate degree in nurse midwifery, and is a fully educated professional specializing in natural childbirth in low-risk patients. She collaborates with a board-certified back-up obstetrician and will either co-manage or refer patients who are not entirely low risk to begin with or develop a problem during pregnancy.

If a woman is interested in a home-like birthing experience, she should choose a midwife and give birth in a hospital birthing room. The birthing room will have a well-equipped hospital and emergency personnel if she needs them and the midwife will have a covering board-certified obstetrician as a back up, should the need arise. Even if she decides that she can do without the pain and chooses to give birth with epidural anesthesia, but would still like a more nurturing, personalized birth experience, she may want to choose a certified nurse midwife. Many CNMs are perfectly willing to deliver patients who choose some type of anesthesia.

A mother can have that kind of experience with many physicians as well, but cannot expect her physician to sit through labor with her, whereas most midwives will be with the mom for the whole time. The nurses on the labor and delivery floor are specialized in supporting women through labor and are generally doing a phenomenal job, but they are strangers that the mom will be meeting for the first time and they could have a personality clash. I recommend that the mom bring her own support system along with her to the hospital, be that the father of the baby, her partner or best friend, a labor coach (doula), or all.

I strongly recommend having a well-trained professional attend to the birth, either a certified nurse-midwife or a physician, preferably an obstetrician/gynecologist. Unless a woman has a family practitioner who delivers a lot of babies, she may be better off with a CNM, who may well be more experienced in childbirth than the family doctor, who occasionally delivers a baby between taking care of sprained ankles, diabetes and high blood pressure.

A further advantage of choosing to deliver a baby in a hospital is that the birthing professional will have been well scrutinized. Only licensed physicians and certified midwifes will have admitting privileges. Their performance, such as number and management of complications, is periodically reviewed and additional supervision and/or training will be imposed on outliers.

There are quite a few marginally trained people out there wanting to deliver babies. Their title and training varies from state to state, as does their licensing status. The medical profession generally refers to them as lay midwives. They vigorously fight this title and want to be called apprentice trained midwives, direct-entry midwifes, professional midwives or licensed midwives, again depending on the state. Their training and diplomas are provided by unregulated institutions that grant their degrees after what I consider only minimal training and experience. It is often impossible for their prospective clients to figure out the legitimacy of their educational claims. As they are not granted hospital privileges, they are the main providers of home births.

I think the most important advice I can give to prospective moms is the following:

- Always keep in mind that the goal is a healthy baby and a healthy mom. There are many ways to achieve that goal.
- Do not get fixated on a specific, inflexible "birthing plan." Choose a hospital that provides birthing rooms and a professional you trust from the list your heath plan provides; then "go with the flow."
- Don't let anyone make you feel guilty about choosing some type of anesthesia. Labor pain is a very individual experience; for some women it is excruciating, while other find it merely uncomfortable. You may find out that "natural childbirth" is not what it is cracked up to be and that you do not take to labor pain like a fish to water. Some people take the boat to Europe and some take a plane. Both get you there. There is no medical evidence that a screaming, hyperventilating mom is better for the baby than a serene mom who can regulate her breathing and focus on her contractions—quite the contrary.
- If a cesarean section becomes necessary, that does not mean that you are a failure. A hundred years ago you might have become a corpse or at least lost your baby. Now a cesarean section is just one more option to help assure your and your baby's safety. And keep in mind that cesarean sections are certainly better than vaginal birth for your pelvic floor muscles and your vagina. There is always a silver lining.

Regula E. Burki, MD, FACOG, is a Board-Certified OB/GYN with a gynecology practice in Salt Lake City, Utah.

WHERE U.S. WOMEN GAVE BIRTH IN 2002

Hospital	99%
Freestanding Birth Center	.29%
Home Birth	.63%
Other	.08%

Source: Center for Disease Control

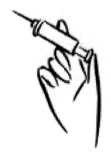

Part Five: Choices Regarding Intervention

Choices Regarding Interventions

It is important to be well informed about all the possible outcomes of labor. By knowing the reasons for all procedures and interventions it is possible to know when they are truly necessary and when one should ask to explore other alternatives.

INTERVENTIONS

by Regula Burki, MD, FACOG

Many different types of interventions are available before and during labor. While birth interventions are seen by some people in this country as negatives, they are responsible for saving the lives of many mothers and babies. Scores of birthing women in developing countries die each year because they have no access to them. The use of some of these interventions may be a matter of preference and comfort to a woman; others may turn out to save her baby's life or brain.

SHOULD I HAVE AN IV DURING LABOR?

An IV is an intravenous line that is placed into one of the veins in the mom's arm. The IV line can either be connected to a bag of intravenous fluid or plugged with a heparin lock right at the level of the skin.

Having an intravenous access during labor is a great advantage should an emergency arise that requires the mom to receive medications rapidly. If she chooses to have her IV plugged, she is not hampered at all in her movements. If the mom needs a continuous infusion of medication, i.e., to make the contractions stronger or an antibiotic to fight infection, the IV, of course, cannot be plugged and will be tethered by a plastic tube to a bag of fluid and medication. The IV bag can be hung on a pole on wheels so the mom can walk around. Moms can generally choose the arm in which to have the IV.

INDUCTION OF LABOR

Induction of labor refers to various methods used to start labor before it starts naturally. It is indicated when the benefit of speeding up the delivery outweighs the risk of continuing the pregnancy. Labor can be induced either by medications or by procedures that stimulate the release of labor-inducing hormones by the body of the pregnant woman.

The statement by Lamaze International printed at page 127 is comprehensive and lists many good references. The most important point it makes is that moms should insist on a clear explanation of why labor is being induced before agreeing to an induction. She should keep asking until all her questions are answered and she understands all the answers!

Drugs to Induce Labor

Pitocin

Pitocin is the brand name for synthetic oxytocin, a hormone that is produced in a gland in the brain and causes the uterus to contract. It is given intravenously to either augment contractions (make them stronger) or to induce labor.

Prostaglandin

Several different prostaglandin preparations are available to ripen (soften) the cervix in preparation for labor or to stimulate contraction of the uterus, either for induction or to stop postpartum hemorrhage. They are administered as gels or suppositories in the vagina, as pills or by injection.

Other Methods for Inducing Labor

Stripping Membranes

The membranes are the bag that contains the amniotic fluid ("water") and the baby. Stripping of the membranes is done by placing a finger in the cervix and gently loosening the membranes from the wall of the uterus around the cervical opening. This can be done wearing sterile gloves during an office visit. It can be quite uncomfortable and generally only works if the body is ready to start labor, such as in women who are overdue. Stripping membranes releases prostaglandins from the cervical tissues and helps soften the cervix.

Rupturing Membranes

Rupturing the membranes means not just loosening the bag of water around the cervix, but actually breaking it. It should be only performed in the hospital under sterile conditions as it is not without risks. It is usually done in combination with other methods of inducing labor.

Intercourse

Intercourse is thought to start contractions by stimulating the cervix and releasing prostaglandins. Like many of the popular methods of starting labor it works best when the body is ready to start labor anyway. Because of the risk of infection, it never should be tried once the bag of water has ruptured on its own but labor has not started yet. That is the time to call the birthing professional and follow her instructions!

Nipple Stimulation

Nipple stimulation releases oxytocin and causes uterine contractions. It can overstimulate the uterus, just as too high a dose of synthetic oxytocin can, and should be done cautiously under the supervision of an experienced birthing professional.

Enema or Eating Spicy Foods

Stimulating the bowels through enemas or eating spicy food is thought to start labor, but probably only works if the mom's body is ready to go into labor anyway. It does, however, have the advantage of keeping the mom from being constipated and in labor at the same time—a definite advantage.

Labor Pain

If the mother finds that the more natural methods of labor pain relief, such as hot showers, massage and breathing, are just not cutting it, there are several methods that are safe for both mom and baby.

Intravenous or Intramuscular Pain Medications

Narcotics given either intravenously or as an intramuscular injection are mostly sedating. They are only effective for labor pain relief in doses so high that they also suppress breathing. Drugs given to mom cross the placenta and affect the baby. If narcotics are given too close before birth, they suppress breathing in the newborn as well. Narcotics also can cause dizziness and nausea. Women who vomit while heavily sedated are at risk of aspirating the contents of their stomachs and getting aspiration pneumonia, which can be life threatening.

Narcotics should be used with caution in laboring women. The use of high doses of narcotics for labor pain relief is not recommended by either the American College of Obstetricians and Gynecologists or the American Society of Anesthesiologists.

Regional Anesthesia

Regional Anesthesia refers to the blocking of sensation below the level of the umbilicus while leaving the mom fully alert. Depending on the medications used for the block, the mom's muscles may function more or less. Some women are able to walk with regional anesthesia. Regional anesthesia is administered by an anesthesiologist either as a spinal or an epidural nerve block, or as a combination of both.

Spinal Nerve Block

With a spinal block, the medication is injected in a single dose directly into the fluid around the spinal cord. The effect is almost immediate and lasts about 30 to 250 minutes depending on the amount of medication used. Because it is a one-time injection, it cannot be prolonged. It is used for the actual delivery of the baby or for cesarean sections, but is not very useful for pain relief during prolonged labor.

Epidural Nerve Block

With an epidural block, a catheter is placed just outside the membrane (dura) that surrounds the spinal cord, allowing for a continuous infusion of medications. The dose and type of medication can be adjusted to the mother's level of pain and rapidly increased should she need emergency surgery.

Combined Spinal Epidural Block

Combined Spinal Epidural anesthesia has the advantage of the rapid onset of pain relief of a spinal and the continuous infusion capability of an epidural. It can be used for a cesarean section and kept for postoperative pain control.

Medications Used for Regional Anesthesia

Long-acting, local anesthetics and narcotics are used either alone or in combination for both spinals and epidurals. The type and dose of drug will be adjusted to the degree of the mother's pain and whether she wants to be able to walk or not.

Possible Problems with Regional Anesthesia

The most annoying problem with an epidural is when it doesn't "take" completely and there is a "window," an area of the mom's body that feels pain while the rest of her lower body is numb! This happens in about 10% of patients and can usually be corrected by administering more or different medication.

The most common side effect of both spinals and epidurals is sudden low blood pressure. To prevent this, the mother will be given extra intravenous fluids before the spinal, but sometimes additional blood pressure boosting medication is necessary. Temporary low blood pressure is not a serious side effect, is treatable and does not hurt the baby.

The next most common side effect is itching when spinal or epidural narcotics are used. Again this can be treated. It is harmless, but annoying and more common with a spinal than with an epidural.

Spinal headache can occur with either spinals or epidurals. Fortunately, it is quite rare (1-2%). It is caused by leakage of spinal fluid through the hole made by the needle injecting the medication. It usually resolves with bed rest, but needs treatment about a third of the time.

Contraindications to Spinal and Epidural Anesthesia

If a woman has a problem with blood clotting, has received blood thinning medications, or has a high fever, she can have neither a spinal nor an epidural.

LOCAL ANESTHESIA

Local anesthesia is generally only used after the delivery to repair any tears around the vaginal opening, or at the time of the delivery to cut an episiotomy. Short-acting anesthetics are generally used.

GENERAL ANESTHESIA

General anesthesia is not used for relief from labor pain, but may be used for an emergency cesarean section when there is no time for a spinal.

FETAL MONITORING

Fetal monitoring refers to checking on the baby's heartbeat during labor and its response to contractions. It can detect normal fetal heart rate changes and changes that signal a problem.

There are two methods of fetal heart rate monitoring. Auscultation is listening to the fetal heartbeat either with a special stethoscope (fetoscope) or a small Doppler ultrasound device through the mother's belly. Electronic fetal monitoring is a procedure in which instruments are used to record the heartbeat of the fetus and the contractions of the mother's uterus during labor. Electronic fetal monitoring can be done either with sensors placed on the mother's abdomen or inside the uterus and on the baby's scalp.

Either auscultation or electronic fetal monitoring can be done at set times during labor or nonstop throughout labor. Which method will be used depends on your risk factors and how labor is progressing.

When electronic fetal monitoring was first developed it was hoped that continuously monitoring the baby's heartbeat was going to be better than intermittent auscultation. Several well conducted studies, however, have shown auscultation is just as good as long as it is done at regular intervals by an experienced nurse who is taking care of only one laboring woman.

OPERATIVE INTERVENTIONS

EPISIOTOMY

When the baby's head is being pushed against the vaginal opening, both by the uterine contractions and the active pushing of the mom, the vaginal tissues get stretched tightly. With repeated pushing, they either stretch to the point that the baby's head can slip through or they rip. An episiotomy is a controlled incision made at the back of the vagina to prevent ragged tearing. If mom does not have an epidural or a spinal, a small amount of local anesthetic is injected before the incision is made. Tearing can also be prevented in the majority of cases if the birthing professional places her hands on the baby's head and guides the baby slowly and carefully through the vaginal opening.

For the greater part of the 20th century, it was believed, especially by American doctors, that episiotomies were necessary to prevent damage to the pelvic tissues and to the baby's head. Many studies have now demonstrated that the routine use of episiotomy did not protect against later dropping of the uterus and bladder or fetal intracranial bleeds. Episiotomy actually increased rates of infection, blood loss, and pain during healing, negatively affecting body image issues and sexual function. It also increased the incidence of injuries to the anal sphincter and the risk of fecal incontinence.

Most birthing professionals now perform episiotomies only when necessary, *i.e.* if the head is out, but the shoulders are stuck; the baby is really large; or the mom's tissues are just too tough or scarred to stretch. Overall, the episiotomy rate has dropped by more than 50% in the last 20 years.

FORCEPS AND VACUUM EXTRACTION

Forceps are two spoon-shaped instruments that are placed in the vagina alongside the baby's head. A vacuum extractor is a suction cup-like device that is attached to the baby's scalp. There is an increased risk of bruising the scalp with this method, but the suction cup sometimes fits better in a tight vagina than the forceps. Both forceps and vacuum extractors are instruments that are applied to the baby's head in order to pull from below, while the mother pushes from above. Both are sometimes used to gently rotate the baby's head if it is not in the optimal position for passing through the birth canal. Both methods should only be used by birthing professionals trained and experienced in their use, which generally means a board certified obstetrician.

Reasons for Forceps Delivery or Vacuum Extraction

In the past, it was believed that if the second stage of labor, the actual pushing phase of the delivery, lasted more than two hours, the risk of the baby dying or sustaining serious damage was greatly increased. Forceps and vacuum extractors were used to pull out the baby before such damage occurred. We now have much more sophisticated methods to identify babies that may not be tolerating labor well and are at risk and the routine, arbitrary use of forceps or vacuum extractor after two hours of pushing is no longer recommended. However, if the mom is completely exhausted, if she has been pushing for two to three hours without making any progress, or if the baby shows signs of fetal distress, either vacuum extraction or forceps delivery is indicated and very safe in experienced hands.

Cautions Regarding Forceps and Vacuum Extraction

Vacuum extraction should not be done and forceps should be used with caution in premature infants and in babies with certain congenital anomalies and blood clotting disorders. Neither should be attempted unless the birthing professional is well trained and experienced in their use and the baby is low enough that the doctor can be sure to deliver the baby vaginally. If that is not the case or if there is any doubt, a cesarean section is safer for both mother and baby.

Cesarean Section

What is a Cesarean Section?

A cesarean section is the surgical delivery of the baby through an abdominal incision. Supposedly, Julius Caesar was delivered in this manner, hence the name.

How is it done? After the skin is thoroughly cleansed with an aseptic solution and sterile drapes spread over the surgical field, the abdomen is entered by making an incision through all layers of the abdominal wall: the skin, the fat, and then several muscle layers and muscle sheaths (fascia). This incision can be made either vertically below the umbilicus like a zipper, or horizontally right above the pubic bone, a "bikini cut." Usually all the intestines have been pushed up into the upper abdomen by the enlarged uterus and the uterus lies directly against the abdominal wall.

Next, the incision through the muscle wall of the uterus is made and stopped just short of the amniotic sac that contains the baby. At this point, everybody gets ready for the arrival of the baby, including dad with the camera. The amniotic sac is ruptured carefully, so as not to hurt the baby, and the baby is delivered much as if she were coming out through the vagina. After the baby is dried and wrapped in soft cloths, the mom can often hold her baby, or at least touch while dad holds the baby. The time from the incision of the skin to the delivery of the baby can be less than three minutes if an emergency requires it, but usually takes about 10 minutes.

If the incision into the uterus is made horizontally in the lower part of the uterus (low transverse incision), the woman is eligible for a trial of labor in a later pregnancy. Rarely, the incision has to be made, or extended, vertically into the upper part of the uterus ("classical" incision) in order to get the baby out. After a classical incision, future labor is too much of a stress for the uterine scar—it will burst and all subsequent pregnancies will have to be delivered by cesarean section. Rupture of the uterus during labor can occur even without a previous cesarean section but it is rare. It is life threatening to both mom and baby. Immediate surgery, however, can save both their lives (another reason not to have a home birth!).

After the baby is delivered, the placenta is removed through the same uterine incision as the baby, and the uterus and abdomen are closed layer by layer in reverse order. This takes about 15 to 20 minutes.

ANESTHESIA FOR CESAREAN SECTIONS

Generally cesarean sections are done under either a spinal or an epidural nerve block. This allows for the mother to be fully conscious and accompanied by a family member or friend.

The mother has, of course, the option to request general anesthesia. The anesthesiologist then waits until the last possible moment before putting the mother under anesthesia, so the baby is still awake by the time he is being delivered. The medications take a few minutes to reach the baby.

The only other time general anesthesia is used is when an acute emergency arises requiring a cesarean section in a woman who does not already have a spinal or an epidural. When minutes can make the difference between life and death, a general anesthetic is usually faster. At such times, the family will not accompany the mother to the operating room, as the nurses and doctors are too busy saving the mom's or the baby's life to have time to instruct lay people on how not to be in the way or contaminate the surgery. Fortunately, such emergencies are rare; but all major labor and delivery floors have an OR ready to go at all times, even while the mother is laboring in a pretty birthing room with lace and ruffles.

REASONS FOR A CESAREAN SECTION

A cesarean delivery should be performed when it is safer for the mother or the baby than a vaginal delivery. That can sometimes be determined before labor and a cesarean section will be scheduled. In this case, it is important to be very sure how far along the pregnancy is, so as not to deliver a baby prematurely.

Here are some examples of reasons for a scheduled cesarean delivery:
- Previous surgery on the uterus, such as removal of fibroids from deep in the muscle wall of the upper part of the uterus, or cesarean section with a high (classical) incision.
- Infectious conditions of the mom that could infect the baby in the birth canal—HIV, large vaginal warts, acute herpes outbreak at the onset of labor.
- Medical conditions of the mom that make labor too great a risk for her, such as extremely high blood pressure or severe diabetes.
- The baby is too big for the size of the mom's pelvis ("cephalopelvic disproportion"). Sometimes this is so obvious that a cesarean delivery

is scheduled from the outset; sometimes the decision is made to do a "trial of labor" and see what happens and only resort to a cesarean delivery when the baby appears to be stuck ("failure to progress in labor").

• More than one baby. Risks are greatly elevated, especially for the second or third baby, because the placenta may detach from the wall of the uterus before all the babies are out.

• The exit is blocked. If a large tumor is located in the lower part of the uterus, it may block passage of the baby through the birth canal. The placenta can cover the cervix and block the exit. This is called placenta praevia.

• The baby is breech. Even though many babies can be delivered in the breech position (bottom first), the risk of complications is greatly increased because the head and shoulders are the largest parts of a newborn. Once they have stretched the birth canal and are out the rest follows automatically. When the smaller bottom end comes out first, the head may get trapped, and the umbilical cord compressed between the baby's skull and the mom's pelvic bones. The baby then does not get any oxygen because the placental blood is cut off and the head is not yet out in the air. The American College of Obstetricians and Gynecologists now recommends that an attempt should be made to turn breech babies in late pregnancy and only deliver them by cesarean section if turning them fails.

• The mom wants a cesarean section. A woman can choose to have a cesarean. She may choose this because she had one before and feels since she already has a scar, she does not want to subject her pelvis and vagina to the trauma of labor. Or she may just decide that labor is not for her (she may have problems to get her insurance company to pay in that case). Even with a previous cesarean women and their doctors have been pressured by the insurance companies to do a "trial of labor" (see section on VBAC).

Sometimes the need for a cesarean section becomes apparent only during labor on a more or less emergency basis. In this case it is irrelevant if the baby is premature or not, as labor is already underway.

Here are some examples of when a cesarean delivery becomes medically advised once labor has started:

• Baby problems, possible fetal distress: During labor the baby's heart rate, including how it responds to contractions, is followed either with a monitor or by auscultation. A non-reassuring fetal heart rate pattern can be a sign that the baby is not receiving enough oxygen. This can occur because the cord is tightly wrapped around the baby's neck or shoulder, the placenta is separating from the uterine wall, or the baby is at risk for some other reason.

- Mom problems: Rarely, laboring women develop medical problems, such as seizures, that make it unsafe for them to continue with labor.
- Placental problems: This usually involves the placenta beginning to separate from the uterine wall (abruption placentae). Signs of this are excessive bleeding and fetal distress.
- Labor problems ("Failure to progress"): About 30% of cesarean deliveries are done for this reason. The most common reason the baby stops advancing down the birth canal is that the baby does not fit ("cephalo-pelvic disproportion"). If labor is allowed to continue indefinitely, something will eventually give—either the baby will develop fetal distress or the uterus will rupture.

Another reason for labor not to progress is that the contractions are not strong enough. If it is early in labor, before the membranes are ruptured, and the baby appears to be comfortable and doing well, there is nothing wrong with just waiting for a while. Usually, before going to a cesarean delivery, augmentation of labor with Pitocin will be attempted.

How important is it to avoid a cesarean section?

My recommendation is that women not obsess over avoiding a cesarean delivery. A mother should pick a birth professional she can trust to carefully explain why a cesarean section has become necessary, should the need for one arise, and then go with her recommendation. It is highly unlikely that an experienced doctor will bully a mother into an unnecessary cesarean section. If the whole prenatal care has been conducted in a "my way or the highway" style, the mom should not be in labor under such a person's care; but if she is, she still should go with the recommendation, because she simply does not have the medical knowledge at that point to determine if her baby's life or brain is at risk or not.

Some things that lead to a cesarean delivery are outside the mother's control; others can be addressed during pregnancy and labor in hopes of lowering the risk of ending up with a cesarean delivery:

Before Labor

- Eat well. Remember that "eating for two" in pregnancy means quality not quantity. You cannot stay healthy and grow a healthy baby on

junk food. Excessive weight gain increases your risk of having a baby too large to fit your pelvis. There are many excellent guidelines on healthy nutrition in pregnancy. Follow them!
• Stay fit or get fit: If you are out of shape, you are ill prepared for a successful labor. Remember that labor means *work*—and it is hard work. Get yourself ready for it.
• Learn as much as you can about what to expect.
• Line up knowledgeable labor support. The last thing you will want to do in labor is explain to your support people what is going on and what you want them to do. Insist that the people you plan to have with you in labor come to prenatal classes with you, or hire a labor coach or doula.
• Pick a good birthing professional you can trust. This does not necessarily mean the doctor with the lowest C-section rate as many factors, such as patient mix, can influence a doctor's section rate. Make sure you pick a doctor or midwife who is willing to answer your questions openly and understandably. Should you end up with a cesarean section, it is crucial that you trust your doctor to be doing the right thing.

During Labor

• Keep moving as long as you can tolerate it. Walking, taking a hot shower, or rocking in a rocking chair lets gravity help guide the baby down in the birth canal and helps you keep your muscles loose. Laying flat on your back does not.
• Try to put off getting an epidural as long as possible. It is not clear from several well-conducted studies that epidurals increase your risk of a cesarean section, but they can certainly slow down your labor, especially if given too early.
• Rest when you can. Labors, especially first labors, can last many hours. You do not want to reach the home stretch when it is finally time to start pushing, totally exhausted. You may be asked to push with every contraction for two or three hours.
• Keep up your energy. Eat and drink at least in early labor, so you have enough energy to last you through to the end.
• Use all the help you can get, be that support people to help you breathe through all your contractions or an epidural when the pain gets to be more than you are willing to endure. Remember that you are the Prima Donna of this event—let them all treat you like one!

VBAC (Vaginal Birth after Cesarean Section)

Partially under the pressure of lawsuits, the cesarean section rate increased from 5% in 1970 to 25% in 1988. Doctors are rarely sued for a poor outcome if they have performed a cesarean section but they are almost always sued when they have not. The courts firmly believed for many years that electronic fetal monitoring could identify practically every baby in trouble and that failure to recognize an abnormal tracing and immediately perform a cesarean section constituted "malpractice" and grounds for several million dollars in payment. Doctors started practicing what is referred to as "defensive medicine" under the rule "when in doubt, section." Women paid with a high rate of often unnecessary cesarean sections. More recent research has shown that fetal monitor tracings are not as failsafe as previously thought and that many serious fetal problems start long before the onset of labor. The practice of "once a cesarean, always a cesarean," which dominated American obstetrics for nearly 70 years, further contributed to the high cesarean delivery rate, as did the fact that more older women with more medical problems and less stretchy tissues began having babies.

In the 1980s, it became clear that sometimes a trial of labor (meaning attempting labor) after a previous cesarean delivery can be safe for carefully selected patients. The National Institute of Health and the American College of Obstetricians and Gynecologists began to encourage the practice for carefully selected women with a low transverse uterine incision. Obviously, when a tiny woman with a small pelvis is expecting another ten-pound baby, the baby will not fit the second time around either!

Unfortunately, many managed care plans proceeded to mandate that all women must have a trial of labor before the insurance company would pay for a cesarean section, and went on a publicity campaign denouncing doctors and hospitals with high cesarean delivery rates. As a result, in many lay circles a doctor's cesarean rate became the sole criteria of competence as an obstetrician!

After 20 years of experience with VBACs, the following points have been shown by several well conducted studies:
- Major complications, such as uterine rupture, surgical complications, and need for hysterectomy, are almost twice as likely with an attempted VBAC as with a scheduled repeat cesarean section.
- The risk of uterine rupture is almost five times higher when VBAC labor is induced with prostaglandins; when induced without prostaglandins the risk is not much higher than that of spontaneous labor.

- Uterine rupture increases the risk of death for the baby ten-fold.
- Depending on how carefully VBAC candidates are selected, in 20-40% of cases the trial of labor fails and the woman ends up with a cesarean section anyway.
- There are no studies showing that VBAC or cesarean delivery is safer for the mother or the baby.
- A successful VBAC has a lower risk of blood transfusion and infection, a shorter hospital stay and shorter postpartum recovery than a repeat cesarean section. It is also cheaper unless the labor was prolonged and complicated.
- A failed VBAC followed by a cesarean section carries a much higher risk of major and minor complications and is more expensive than a scheduled repeat cesarean section.
- The American College of Obstetricians and Gynecologists advises that most women with one or two low-transverse uterine incisions from a previous cesarean delivery who have no contraindications for vaginal birth are candidates for an attempted VBAC. The risk of uterine rupture increases with the number of previous uterine incisions. VBAC should be tried only if a physician capable of performing an emergency cesarean section is immediately available to monitor the entire active phase of labor. The mother should be in a hospital with an in-house anesthesiologist and operating room personnel.
- No women should be bullied into a VBAC by her peers, her midwife, her doctor or her insurance plan.

The foregoing was written by Regula Burki, MD, FACOG.

RECOMMENDATIONS FROM LAMAZE INTERNATIONAL

Lamaze International recommends that pregnant women neither choose nor agree to be induced unless there is a true medical indication for induction. A pregnant woman in a Lamaze class told the class, "My doctor says the baby is pretty big. He recommends that I be induced after I reach 38 weeks."

All over the United States, similar statements are heard in childbirth classes. Elective induction of labor is the most controversial issue in maternity care today. In many hospitals, induction of labor is only done for medical reasons. Strict guidelines are adhered to. However, in many other hospitals, almost all women today are induced. Why the differences? Are there problems with induction?

What Is Induction?

Induction is the artificial initiation of labor. Most commonly, labor is induced in the hospital setting by administering the drug pitocin through an IV. Sometimes ripening agents are used in advance to soften and prepare the cervix for labor.

Medical Indications for Induction

There are good medical reasons to induce labor. According to the American College of Obstetricians and Gynecologists, labor should be induced only when it is more risky for the baby to remain inside the mother's uterus than to be born. This is true when the bag of water breaks and labor does not begin; when the pregnancy has reached 42 weeks; when the mom's blood pressure is high; when the mom has other health problems that can harm the baby such as diabetes or lung disease; or when she has an infection of the uterus.[1]

Having a large or very large baby is not listed as one of the medical indications for induction by the American College of Obstetricians and Gynecologists. In fact, a study published in a 1997 edition of the *Journal of Maternal-Fetal Medicine* indicated that induction for macrosomia (large baby) increases rather than decreases cesarean section rates.[2] In the professional publication *Evaluation of Cesarean Delivery* published by the American College of Obstetricians and Gynecologists in 2000, the authors recommend against induction for large babies in healthy women, concluding that, "Induction of labor for suspected macrosomia [large baby] does not improve outcome, expends considerable resources, and may increase the cesarean delivery rate."[3]

Other Reasons for Induction

In addition to the benefits of induction to the health of the mother and baby when medically indicated, induction is often convenient for everyone involved. Hospitals can staff extra nurses during shifts when inductions are scheduled; physicians can schedule births for the days and hours that are most convenient for them; and expectant parents can arrange work and travel arrangements for relatives according to the scheduled date of induction.

Disadvantages of Induction

There is growing evidence that elective induction of labor (induction that is done for convenience rather than for one of the medical indications) is not a risk-free procedure. For one thing, due dates are not always exact. If there is a two week error in calculating the due date, a woman scheduled to be induced for convenience at 38 weeks might be only 36 weeks pregnant.

Dr. Michael Kramer of McGill University in Montreal and his colleagues examined 4.5 million births in the United States and Canada during the 1990s. In a study published in the August 2000 edition of *The Journal of the American Medical Association (JAMA)*, the researchers concluded that babies born only a few weeks early—at 34 weeks through 36 weeks—were nearly three times more likely to die in their first year of life than full-term infants.[4] "Obstetricians may perceive the induction as risk-free and therefore not adequately balance the risks and benefits," Dr. Kramer said in a later interview.

Researchers at the prestigious Southwestern Medical School in Dallas, Texas also recently looked at pregnancy outcomes by week of gestation. After examining more than 56,000 pregnancy outcomes at 40, 41, and 42 weeks, Dr. James Alexander and his fellow researchers concluded that, "Routine labor induction at 41 weeks likely increases labor complications and operative delivery without significantly improving neonatal outcomes."[5] Their recommendation is that physicians not induce a post-term pregnancy until the pregnancy reaches 42 weeks.

Need for Increased Interventions

In addition to the increased risks of mild prematurity and the increased risk of cesarean birth, an induced labor often creates the need for additional medical interventions. In many cases, if a mom is induced, she will require an IV and continuous electronic fetal heart rate monitoring.

In many settings, the mother will be required to stay in bed or very close to the bed. She may be unable to walk freely or to change positions in response to labor contractions, both of which may help labor to progress. She may be unable to take advantage of a soothing tub bath or a warm shower to ease the pain of labor contractions. Artificially induced contractions often peak sooner and remain intense longer than natural contractions, increasing her need for pain medications.

Psychological Disadvantage

Inducing labor, especially when not medically indicated, can give you a powerful message that the mother's body is not working correctly—that she need help to begin labor. This message along with the increased need for medical interventions may decrease her confidence in her ability to give birth.

The Recommendation of Lamaze International

Lamaze International recommends that a mother neither choose nor agree to be induced unless there is a true medical indication for induction. A "large" or even "very large" baby is not a medical indication for induction in the nondiabetic woman. Allowing the mother's body to go into labor spontaneously almost always is the best indication that the baby is ready to be born. Experiencing natural contractions produced by the mother's own body's oxytocin increases the freedom that she has to be able to respond to contractions by moving around, changing positions, and trying the tub or shower. Laboring and giving birth without unnecessary medical intervention increases the likelihood that she will have positive lifelong memories of her birth experience and decreases the possibilities of complications to both her and the baby.

1. American College of Obstetricians and Gynecologists (ACOG) (2000), *Planning Your Pregnancy and Birth*, Washington, DC: ACOG.
2. Leaphart, W.L., Meyer, M.C. & Capeless, E.L. (1997). "Labor Induction with a Prenatal Diagnosis of Fetal Macrosomia," *The Journal of Maternal-Fetal Medicine, 6* (2), 99-102.
3. American College of Obstetricians and Gynecologists (ACOG) (2000), *Evaluation of Cesarean Delivery*, Washington, DC: ACOG.
4. Kramer, M.S., et al. (2000). "The Contribution of Mild and Moderate Preterm Birth to Infant Mortality," *JAMA, 284* (7), 843-849.
5. Alexander, J.M., McIntire, D.D., & Leveno, K.J. (2000), "Forty Weeks and Beyond: Pregnancy Outcomes by Week of Gestation," *Obstetrics & Gynecology, 96* (2), 291-294.

Reprinted with the permission of Lamaze International.
www.lamaze.org
1-800-368-4404

Things You Can Do To Avoid an Unnecessary Cesarean Section
from the International Cesarean Awareness Network

The Public Citizen Health Research Group in Washington, D.C. has estimated that half of the nearly one million cesareans performed every year are medically unnecessary. With more appropriate care during pregnancy, labor, and delivery, half of the cesareans could have been avoided. Clearly there are times when cesareans are necessary. However, cesareans increase the risk to both mothers and babies. These are suggestions for things you can do to avoid an unnecessary cesarean and help insure that your birth experience is as healthy and positive as possible.

Before Labor
- Read and educate yourself; attend classes and workshops inside and outside the hospital.
- Research and prepare a birth plan. Discuss your birth plan with your midwife or doctor and submit copies to your hospital or birth center.
- Interview more than one care provider. Ask key questions and see how your probing influences their attitude. Are they defensive or pleased by your interest?
- Ask your care provider if there is a set time limit for labor and second stage pushing. See what they feel can interfere with the normal process of labor.
- Tour more than one birth facility. Note their differences and ask about their cesarean rate, VBAC protocol, etc.
- Become aware of your rights as a pregnant woman.
- Find a labor support person. Interview more than one. A recent medical journal article showed that labor support can significantly reduce the risk of cesarean.
- Help ensure a healthy baby and mother by eating a well-balanced diet.
- If your baby is breech, ask your care provider about exercises to turn the baby, external version (turning the baby with hands), and vaginal breech delivery. You may want to seek a second opinion.
- If you had a cesarean, seriously consider VBAC. According to the American College of Obstetricians & Gynecologists, VBAC is safer in most cases than a scheduled repeat cesarean and up to 80% of

woman with prior cesareans can go on to birth their subsequent babies vaginally.

DURING LABOR
- Stay at home as long as possible. Walk and change positions frequently. Labor in the position most comfortable for you.
- Continue to eat and drink lightly, especially during early labor, to provide energy.
- Avoid pitocin augmentation for a slow labor. As an alternative, you may want to try nipple stimulation.
- If your bag of water breaks, don't let anyone do a vaginal examination unless medically indicated for a specific reason. The risk of infection increases with each examination. Discuss with your care provider how to monitor for signs of infection.
- Request intermittent electronic fetal monitoring or the use of a fetoscope. Medical research has shown that continuous electronic fetal monitoring can increase the risk of cesarean without related improvement in outcome for the baby.
- Avoid using an epidural. Medical research has shown that epidurals can slow down labor and cause complications for the mother and baby. If you do have an epidural and have trouble pushing, ask to take a break from pushing until the epidural has worn off some and then resume pushing.
- Do not arrive at the hospital too early. If you are still in the early stages of labor when you get to the hospital, instead of being admitted, walk around the hospital or go home and rest.
- Find out the risks and benefits of routine and emergency procedures before you are faced with them. When faced with any procedure, find out why it it's being used in your case, what are the short and long term effects on you and your baby, and what are your other options.
- Remember, nothing is absolute. If you have doubts, trust your instincts. Do not be afraid to assert yourself. Accept responsibility for your requests and decisions.

Information reprinted with the permission of International Cesarean Awareness Network.

Part Six: Choices Regarding Birth Environment and Managing Labor

Choices Regarding Birth Environment and Managing Labor

One of the great things about giving birth now, rather than in previous decades, is the increased control we have over the birth environment. Many of us who are in our 30s or 40s ask our mothers about their birth experiences, and they answer that they don't remember. They were rendered unconscious and wheeled into what was essentially an operating room. Fathers waited outside.

Today, we can choose where and how we give birth. We can choose whom we want to be present (and whom we don't!) and, to a certain extent, what we want to hear and smell. We can choose to stand, walk, squat, or lie down, and how we want to be touched (or not touched!).

Of course, all of your wishes may not come true; some may need to be set aside in the interests of a healthy baby, the ultimate goal, but it doesn't hurt to wish.

Who Present

One of the most important decisions you will make is whom you want present during the birth. Most woman want their birth partner or other labor coach present, but you may also want relatives and children present (though it may be too scary for children under the age of ten or twelve). Some women choose to bring in their own pediatric or obstetrical nurse as well.

The people you choose to be present must be chosen well. You must have complete confidence in them to be supportive, fulfill your birth plan to the extent possible, and shield you from outside distractions. You might choose someone specifically to be the gatekeeper and make sure no unauthorized people, either personally or by phone, intrude on the labor and delivery. You should also let people know before labor that no uninvited guests will be allowed in.

Handling Inquiries

You might want to choose a reliable, tactful, trusted family member to handle inquiries (usually phone calls) from family and friends wondering about the progression of the labor and delivery. (One mom-to-be got a conference call from the law firm where she worked put through to the delivery room. The firm had called her to give her a chance to argue her case for maternity leave. She was 10 hours into labor. She took the call, hung up and was so angry, she dilated to 10 and immediately delivered. This method is NOT recommended!) The Gatekeeper (or Information Officer) needs to have tact: the ability to be discreet if the labor, delivery, or status of the newborn is problematic, and also understanding of the concerns of family and friends. Preferably, this will be a person known to friends and family members, not someone who appears to be a stranger keeping them from knowing the condition of their loved ones.

What Props?

Women can take all kinds of comfort items into their labor room: music, candles, scents, favorite pillows or throws, pictures, a talisman, favorite massage oil, poetry books, hard candy, juices—all packed in the overnight bag or set up in anticipation of a home birth.

Birthing Positions

by Paulina G. Perez, RN, BSN, FACCE, CD

Fortunately, we've left behind the days of the laboring-on-her-back, heavily sedated mother-to-be, totally dissociated from the natural workings of her own body and missing out on the joy of giving birth.

Today, women can learn how to use their bodies to minimize discomfort and speed the progress of labor. Trying a variety of positions during labor and birth can help you find what works best for you. Here is what you need to know about the various labor and birth positions.

Standing

Advantages
- Excellent for oxygenation of fetus
- Uses gravity
- Contractions are more effective and less painful
- Helps speed up labor; helps create pushing urge

Disadvantages
- Poor control of delivery
- Visualization very hard for birth attendant

Walking

Advantages
- Uses gravity
- Contractions often less painful
- Encourages uterine contractility
- Baby well aligned in pelvis
- May speed up labor
- Reduces backache; encourages descent

Disadvantages
- Often mother can't use if she has high blood pressure
- Can't be used with continuous electronic fetal monitoring

Sitting

Advantages
- Good for resting
- Uses gravity
- Can be used with continuous electronic monitoring
- Can be used with birth ball to encourage descent

Disadvantages
- Possibly can't be used if mother has high blood pressure

Sitting on Toilet

Advantages
- Helps relax perineum
- Mother accustomed to open-leg position and pelvic pressure in this environment
- Uses gravity

Disadvantages
- Pressure from toilet seat can cause pain

Semi-Sitting

Advantages
- Good use of gravity
- Good resting position
- Works well in hospital beds
- Good visibility at delivery for the mom, dad and others present
- Good access to FHTs (Fetal Heart Tones)

Disadvantages
- Access to perineum can be poor
- Mobility of coccyx is impaired
- Some stress on perineum, but less than lithotomy

LITHOTOMY (ON BACK, LEGS RAISED — AVOID THIS POSITION!)
Disadvantages
- Compression of all major vessels
- Laceration or need for episiotomy is more likely
- No use of gravity to aid delivery

SIDE-LYING
Advantages
- Good fetal oxygenation
- Good resting position for mother
- Helpful if mother has elevated blood pressure
- Useful if mother has epidural anesthesia
- Often makes contractions more effective
- May promote progress of labor
- Easier for the mom to relax between contractions during second stage
- Allows posterior sacral movement in second stage
- Can slow precipitous delivery
- Partner can support mother's leg
- Partner can assist in delivery
- Lowers chance of laceration or need for episiotomy
- Access to perineum is excellent

Disadvantages
- Access to FHTs poor if mother is lying on same side as baby's back
- No help from gravity
- Mother must support her leg under knee if no one is there to hold leg
- Mother may feel too passive

LEANING
Advantages
- Great for rotation of posterior presentation
- Uses gravity

- Contractions often less painful
- Contractions often more productive
- Baby is well aligned in pelvis
- Relieves backache
- Facilitates use of back pressure
- May be more restful than standing

Disadvantages
- Hard for attendant if used at delivery

KNEELING, LEANING FORWARD WITH SUPPORT
Advantages
- Helpful with persistent posterior presentation
- Assists rotation of baby
- Good for pelvic rocking
- Good for use with birth ball
- Less strain on wrists and arms

SQUATTING
Advantages
- Encourages rapid descent
- Uses gravity
- May increase rotation of baby
- Allows freedom to shift weight for comfort
- Excellent for access to the perineum
- Excellent for fetal circulation
- May increase pelvis diameter by as much as two centimeters
- Requires less bearing-down effort
- Upper trunk presses on fundus to encourage descent
- Thighs keep baby well aligned

Disadvantages
- Often tiring to the mother
- Sometimes hard to hear FHTs
- May be hard for the mother to assist in delivery

HANDS AND KNEES
Advantages
- Good for bradycardia (low heart tones)
- Good for back labor

- Useful with birth ball
- Assists with rotation of posterior presentation
- Takes pressure off hemorrhoids
- Best position to avoid laceration or need for episiotomy
- Good delivery position for large baby
- Excellent for shoulder dystocia

Disadvantages
- Hard to maintain eye contact with mother
- Hard for mother to see
- Baby must be passed through mother's legs
- Can be disorienting to inexperienced attendant.

Reprinted with the permission of Paulina G. (Polly) Perez, RN, BSN, LCCE, FACCE, president of C.F.E., Inc., in Johnson, VT and a perinatal nurse consultant, doula trainer and monitrice in private practice. (A monitrice is a labor assistant who provides emotional and physical support and has the ability to clinically assess both mother and baby.)

BIRTH BALLS

by Paulina G. Perez, RN, BSN, FACCE, CD

I first encountered this labor tool over ten years ago while on a trip to Europe. While there, I visited several people who had told me to look them up if I ever got to Germany, so I took them up on their offer. One of them wanted me to see the hospital where she had birthed her first baby, so a trip to her local hospital was in store.

My journey learning about the "birth ball" was about to begin. I visited a labor ward while I was in Germany. It was quite standard, as labor wards go, except that in the first room they showed me there was a huge ball. I was still in the dark, so I asked them to demonstrate what they did with the ball. I was shown positions to use to help the baby descend into the pelvis and also to help the baby rotate. When I got home, I got one immediately and started using it in both my childbirth education and labor support practice. The more I used it, the more uses I found for it. The appropriate size of ball is determined by the height of the woman using it. Women under 5'2" should use a 53 cm ball; those 5' 2" - 5' 7" should use a 65 cm ball; and women over 5' 7" should use a 75 cm ball.

How the Ball is Used

"Birth balls" promote optimal positioning and pain reduction during contractions and also elicit *spontaneous, non-habituating movement*. This spontaneous gentle movement is part of the reason the birth ball works so effectively in labor. The ball needs to move freely so that the mother does not habituate to one position.

The ball can also be used effectively with electronic fetal monitoring. It encourages fetal descent as the mother remains sitting in an upright posture, taking advantage of gravity while keeping the fetus well aligned in the pelvis.

1. Hold the ball with your hand as you sit down on it with your feet flat on the floor and about two feet apart to give you a stable base.
2. If the mother is concerned about feeling stable, have her partner, professional labor assistant, nurse or midwife stand behind her until she feels stable.
3. Use of the ball is demonstrated by Paulina Perez, Penny Simkin and other trainers in doula workshops throughout North America, as well as in the videos *Special Women: How A Labor Assistant Makes Birth Safe, Satisfying and Less Costly* and *Comfort Measures for Childbirth* by Penny Simkin. Both videos are available from Cutting Edge Press.

Why Use This Ball?

1. In the last month of pregnancy, pregnant women find it easier than a chair or couch to get up and down from.
2. It encourages pelvic mobility.
3. It allows the mother the freedom to rock her pelvis, change her position and shift her weight for comfort.
4. It encourages fetal descent as the mother remains sitting in an upright posture, taking advantage of gravity.
5. Sitting on the ball helps keep the fetus well aligned in the pelvis.
6. The ball encourages pelvic relaxation by conforming to the mother's body similar to a water mattress as it provides perineal support without undue pressure.
7. Sitting on warm compresses on the ball will maximize perineal relaxation.
8. Sitting on the ball encourages rhythmic movement as the mother sways or rocks back and forth while sitting on the ball.
9. Sitting on the ball while leaning over the bed gives the mother the

pelvic mobility that she is unable to have while sitting on a chair.
10. Less strain on the hands and arms when mother is in the hands and knees position.
11. Eliminates hard external pressure of a chair, bed or rocker when sitting.
12. May speed up labor.
13. Can be used as a support while squatting so that the ball presses on the fundus to encourage fetal descent. Squatting helps widen pelvic outlet to its maximum.
14. Its use is beneficial with techniques for "failure to progress."
15. Ball use is also helpful for strengthening lower back for those with chronic back pain.
16. Ball use can also strengthen abdominal muscles used in second stage labor.

Use in Back Labor or Persistent Posterior Fetal Position

1. Having the mother lean over the ball while on her hands and knees gives her good pelvic mobility, as well as uses gravity to encourage the largest and heaviest part of the baby's body to rotate.
2. Kneeling and leaning over the ball assists in rotation of the baby to the anterior.
3. As the mother's weight is totally supported by the birth ball, she is able to stay in the critical hands and knees position for an extended length of time. Normally, the mother is only able to maintain this position for a short interval as it causes carpal tunnel syndrome by putting excess strain on her wrists and hands and is tiring as she must support her entire body weight.
4. The use of the ball has saved more than a few mothers from a cesarean section for failure to progress.
5. It is easier for someone to do counterpressure for the mother's back pain while in the hands and knees position over the ball.

Ball Use in the Postpartum Period

1. With a fussy baby, simply sit on the ball and sway or bounce slightly while patting the baby. The mother should always steady the ball when the baby is on it.
2. Mothers also report that they have used it for colic by placing the baby on its stomach on it; the pressure on the baby's abdomen seems to help.

3. Exercises using the ball in the postpartum period can help firm and tone the hip and buttocks, inner and outer thighs and abdomen. Postpartum exercises for the lower body are explained in detail in *The Body Ball Book*, available from Cutting Edge Press.

COMMENTS FROM MOTHERS WHO HAVE USED THE BALL

Utah—"I leaned over it and did pelvic rocks to help my baby turn."
Arizona—"I couldn't have dealt with my induction of labor without it."
Texas—"I sat on it and leaned over the bed the whole time I was in labor. I'm not sure what I would have done without it."
California—"It sure helped my baby to turn; I loved it."
Missouri—"My midwife said that without it I might have had to have a cesarean."

COMMENTS FROM NURSES, MIDWIVES AND PROFESSIONAL LABOR ASSISTANTS WHO USE THE BALL

Vermont—"I use it all the time now."
Texas—"I never attend a birth without it."
California—"My clients love it."
Florida—"I demonstrate it in my childbirth classes and encourage moms to use it."
Indiana—"It gives me one more tool to use for those moms with back labor."
Maryland—"Our hospital has them in all the labor rooms."

The 65-cm ball is available from Cutting Edge Press, along with ball covers and carrying straps. Also check the photos at http://childbirth.org/CEP/ballhow.html

The uses for the balls are covered in the book Birth Balls: The Use of Physical Therapy Balls in Maternity Care by Paulina Perez, RN. The book also contains valuable tips from doulas, nurses, midwives and childbirth educators. This book is available at Cutting Edge Press (www.birthballs.com) and Amazon.com and is the only book about the use of physical therapy balls in maternity care. The "Gymnastik Birth Ball" is available from Cutting Edge Press. You may reach them by calling 802/635-2142. Cutting Edge Press is also on the Internet at www.birthballs.com or via e-mail at pollyp@pwshift.com.

Managing Labor

Relaxation and Childbirth

by Mary Paliescheskey, BS

Relaxation is the key to handling the increasing intensity of labor. After a contraction has passed, it is very important to let the tension go. Holding tension or anticipating the arrival of the next contraction takes a lot of energy. It can make labor seem more intense and difficult.

Practice relaxation techniques before labor. Deep slow breaths for as long as possible during labor will help keep you relaxed and focused. As labor intensifies, include moaning or toning sounds from deep in the chest (from the diaphragm). Physical touching, massage, holding through contractions, and counter pressure help keep a woman focused and relaxed. Eye contact is especially important. Also use visualization or focal points if they help you maintain a focus. Some women work best by going within themselves. Do not disturb this focus if it's working.

During labor, make sure that your physical needs are met. You need to keep your energy available to you. Food and water can be very important keys to relaxation. If you become dehydrated, you will not be able to handle the intensity of labor. Always drink plenty of water. It is best to drink something every 10-15 minutes. Also, frequent urination is a must—at least once every hour as a full bladder will inhibit the baby from moving through the birth canal. Changing positions and allowing gravity to assist the progress of labor is another important physical need. Spend a good portion of each hour in activity. If labor is long, rest as you can. Support people should keep an eye on the physical needs. Women in labor should live in the moment. Each contraction should be all that matters.

Several relaxation techniques are commonly used in labor: deep breathing, visualization, meditation, music, subdued lighting, shower or tub, and massage. However, your choices are not limited to these. If something isn't working for you, try something else. Other options could include aromatherapy, acupuncture, or anything else that provides comfort and relaxes you.

The most important element in relaxation is creating a safe and supportive environment. The main support person should keep things positive. Avoid all negative comments as they are counter productive. The following are a few examples of supportive and positive statements to use during labor: "You are doing wonderfully. You are so strong. I know things are getting harder, but you can do this. I'm so proud of you." Encourage her that things are progressing well, even if it's slower than she thought it should be. Reassure her that you are there for her and support her choices. Labor happens in its own time.

A sense of safety is very important in labor. If you feel insecure in your surroundings, your body will produce stress hormones that will inhibit the natural process of labor. Relaxation is secondary to a feeling of security and support.

After you feel safe, you can then relax in your birth. Relaxation is the feeling of trust in the birth process. The tools that you use to reach that state are your choice.

From Mothering the Mother Newsletter, reprinted with permission.

COPING WITH LABOR

by Mary Paliescheskey, BS

As a doula and childbirth educator, I find that the burning question in all couples' minds is, "How do I cope with labor?" I will try to answer that question here.

BREATHING

First and foremost is your breath. Breathing is one of the most important aspects of labor. There are basically two breaths for labor: deep, slow breathing and shallow breathing.

Do you need a pattern? Do you need to memorize what breath goes where? Do you need a special breath for each stage of labor? Do you need hypnobirthing or other structured breathing patterns? The answer is a resounding NO.

Can you have great benefits from these programs? Will they help you? Of course. Anything you practice and have faith in will help you.

Breathing during labor is very important. ... You breathe to bring relaxation to your body. You breathe to bring oxygen to your baby and your muscles. Most importantly, you do this to keep your baby healthy through labor, and so that you feel less pain. You do all this by keeping your muscles relaxed.

Your breath is the key to your relaxation. While it is similar to breathing that you do during athletic events, it's not totally the same.

Practice relaxing your muscles. Imagine a contraction building, and practice breathing while relaxing all your other muscles.

You can practice with ice. You hold an ice cube for 60 seconds. Focus on your breath as it moves in and out of your body. Another focus is to listen and/or observe everything in the room except the ice. Another way is to use distraction: read a book or watch TV.

I cannot overemphasize the need for you to practice. I understand that everyone is busy. However, the practice is important in teaching your body to relax around the contraction of your uterus. Your uterus is contracting with increasing intensity. A common reaction to this intensity is to contract other muscles in your body in response. Your shoulders tighten and rise. Your jaw might clench. Practice before your labor will help you cope.

PRACTICE, PRACTICE, PRACTICE

Partners need to practice, too. They need to know how to relax and calm themselves, as well as how to help mom. Partners' emotions have an impact on the laboring mother, so partners need to keep an eye on themselves as well as on mom.

WATER AND FOOD

Hydration is also very important in your ability to cope with the increasing intensity of labor. Drink like you are running a marathon. Keep drinking. Keep the fluid going in your body.

Keeping your body hydrated will keep you feeling better. Dehydration affects not only your perception of pain, but the functioning of your muscles. Dehydration can result in contractions that have no effect on your cervix. You feel the contraction. You work through it. It costs you energy, focus, coping skills. All for nothing if you have become dehydrated.

Therefore, drinking becomes a major coping technique. Water and juice are good choices. Juice not only hydrates you, but gives you some energy as well.

Food is very important in the latent phase of labor (0-4 cm). It is very important to keep your energy levels up. Eat light food. You don't know how long this phase of labor will last.

During active labor, your digestion will shut down. So when you stop wanting food in active labor, listen to your body. Active labor generally moves along at one centimeter an hour, so soon enough, you will get to eat again.

Support

Emotional support during labor is very important. No matter how confident you are in your abilities, it is very important to have people giving you positive feedback.

Support can be very difficult for loved ones to give, not because they don't want to give it, but because watching you move through this difficult process is hard. They feel that they are not doing anything, when the support that they give you cannot be replaced. Without it you would lose your way.

Labor requires concentration and flexibility. Support people are there to monitor the progress. They have little to do as long as the mom remains in the moment, relaxed, and breathing. Their role becomes essential when the mom's concentration breaks down due to long hours and intensity. A support person gets you back to relaxing and breathing.

A support person's main job is to wait in nurturing support. They mirror to the laboring woman how well she is doing. They suggest different positions or relaxation techniques. They keep track of hydration and bathroom breaks—one per hour.

Conclusion

There are many techniques to help you cope with labor, but it ultimately comes down to flexibility. You need to live in the moment. Move through one contraction at a time. No one can birth this baby but you. Have faith that you will have the best birth that you can with the labor that you find yourself in. Every birth is different.

May your journey to family be filled with joy.

Mary Paliescheskey, BS, is an experienced Birth Guide and mother. She holds a Bachelor's of Science Degree in Medical Microbiology from the University of California, Davis and has published in medical journals. She founded Mothering the Mother Birth Services in 1995 to guide women and their partners through the transition of birth. Mothering the Mother is dedicated to assisting families in making informed choices that are best for them. The newsletter is dedicated to the exploration of the choices available for pregnancy, childbirth, and parenting.

For more information contact
Mary Paliescheskey, BS, Birth Guide

617 15th St.
Huntington Beach, CA 92648
http://members.tripod.com/doula
(530) 758-4265

Information reprinted with permission of Mothering the Mother Newsletter.

PREGNANCY AND LABOR GUIDELINES FROM AN OB/GYN

by Jennifer Normoyle, MD, OB/GYN

Childbirth is never easy, but there are women for whom the delivery process is relatively more manageable and who report a positive and fulfilling experience. Maybe there is an element of luck when this occurs, but if so, luck plays only a small part. An "easier" labor is much more likely if you are prepared and trusting of the birth process, are able to maintain a state of relative relaxation during labor, are in a state of good physical fitness, and are well informed as well as well supported. Fifteen specific techniques for achieving these goals include the following:

During Pregnancy

1. MAKE PHYSICAL FITNESS A PRIORITY

Benefits of moderate exercise during pregnancy include fewer backaches, better digestion and less constipation, improved circulation (thus helping to prevent fluid retention and varicose veins), lower stress levels, increased energy levels and enhanced emotional well-being. Women who exercise during pregnancy also have a better body image and are less likely to gain excessive weight. Exercise may also protect against the development of diabetes during pregnancy.

Specific benefits with regards to the labor process include improved endurance and better muscle tone to aid in delivery as well as recovery after birth. Women who exercise during pregnancy have shorter labors with fewer medical and physical interventions.

It's best to initiate regular exercise even before you become pregnant. However, if you are in good health and are having no problems, you can still begin a reasonable exercise program, such as walking or swimming, during pregnancy. Prenatal yoga is an excellent choice for maintaining physical fitness during pregnancy, since it also incorporates breathing and relaxation techniques.

Discuss any specific pregnancy-related modifications that you need to consider while exercising with your doctor or midwife.

2. TAKE A CHILDBIRTH PREPARATION CLASS

Do this by about the seventh month of pregnancy in order to familiarize yourself with the stages of labor and the complications that can occur during childbirth. Understanding what is going on and what to expect decreases fear. In addition, during childbirth classes, relaxation, breathing and visualization techniques are taught to further minimize the anxiety. This, in turn, reduces the production of stress hormones that otherwise make contractions more painful and less effective.

A discussion of medications that can be used during labor is an important part of childbirth preparation classes so that you better understand your options should uncontrollable factors, such as the intensity of the contractions, the position of the baby, or the size and shape of the birth canal, result in a longer, more difficult birth.

In general, it's best to choose a class that your health care provider recommends, since the ideas you learn will be more likely to be in tune with his or her philosophy and practice. Look for a class that minimizes rigid rules, that teaches a variety of comfort techniques and that emphasizes reliance on the laboring woman's own internal cues to guide what strategies are going to work best for her during labor. Smaller classes are preferable, as they allow for more individual attention and stronger camaraderie among the participants.

3. PRACTICE

Even though they seem deceptively simple, practice, practice, practice and then practice some more the relaxation, breathing and visualization techniques learned in your childbirth classes. Try to set at least 15-20 minutes a day or more to do so. With practice, your faith and trust in these techniques will increase and you will more successfully use them during labor.

4. POSITIVE AFFIRMATIONS

Consider the use of positive affirmations during pregnancy to help combat anxiety and fear about labor. An affirmation is a statement about a state of mind that you wish to develop (such as more confidence) or a situation you would like to bring about. Repeated frequently, positive affirmations can help you overcome negative thought patterns (usually compounded by horror tales passed on by well-meaning friends and

relatives) and make your goal of a satisfying birth experience a reality. The best time to use an affirmation is any time you choose. The affirmations you use should be short, simple and meaningful to you. They will be more beneficial if stated with feeling, energy and belief. Example include:
"Giving birth is a normal, healthy event."
"I take responsibility to prepare for my birth wisely."
"I am helping to create a safe, healthy birth for myself and my baby."
"I can flow with labor, my mind in perfect harmony with my body and with nature."

Change the wording of the above suggestions or create your own affirmations to best suit your needs.

5. ENLIST SUPPORT

Constant companionship provided by your partner and/or trusted friends or relatives is essential during the labor and birth experience. Childbirth is not a spectator sport and whoever is present with you during the process should be willing to attend childbirth classes and educate him or herself along with you so that they may more fully and effectively assist you in negotiating the birth process. All of your childbirth companions should have the capacity to be supportive without being insistent and must try to listen to and be in tune with you during labor. They should be able to anticipate your needs and be willing to be perfect servants—available to hold your hand, feed you ice chips, mop your brow, massage your back or neck and help you breathe through your contractions. They should be able to let you be in control, but be able to use simple, direct instructions to help you stay relaxed and focused.

Consider the option of hiring a doula, an individual specifically trained to support a laboring woman and her partner. According to a study published in the May 1999 *American Journal of Obstetrics and Gynecology*, women who had continuous labor care provided by a doula were 30 percent less likely to need pain medication, 50 percent less likely to require cesarean delivery and their labors were 25 percent shorter than those without this care. If you hire a doula, make sure you meet with her well ahead of time and that you feel comfortable with her.

6. Take a tour of the facility where you will deliver

This gives you the opportunity to familiarize yourself with the surroundings and the personnel, and to make sure it provides an environment you feel confidence in for your birth experience.

7. Communication

Talk to your doctor or midwife about specific areas of concern you have and consider putting together a birth "plan" or "wish list" to clarify your preferences about such issues as the use of medications, intravenous fluids, episiotomies, etc. This will help you clarify your thoughts about how you hope your childbirth experience will unfold and will increase your sense of control (keeping in mind that when all is said and done, it may be impossible to have everything go exactly as you wish during labor due to the variety of unforeseen circumstances that are possible).

8. Perineal massage

Consider perineal massage for a few minutes every day or so in the last several weeks of pregnancy. Your perineum is the area between the vagina and the rectum. This kind of massage will prepare you for the sensations of stretching that you will feel during birth and may reduce your need for an episiotomy, as well as possibly reducing the risk of tearing. To do perineal massage, wash your hands and then lubricate your thumbs and perineum with vegetable oil, KY jelly or vitamin E oil. Place your thumbs about an inch or so inside the vagina, then press down and to the sides at the same time. Gently and firmly stretch the skin until you feel a slight tingling or burning sensation. Continue to hold this pressure for an additional two minutes or so until the perineum becomes more numb and the tingling is not as distinct. Then pulling gently outwards or forwards, massage the lower part of the vagina with your thumbs. This massaging motion helps to stretch the perineal skin similar to the way that your baby's head will stretch it during labor.

During Labor

9. Distraction

In early labor, when contractions are relatively mild, engage in distracting activities such as taking a walk, baking cookies, playing cards or listening to soothing music. Slow, deep breathing will help you stay calm, but don't automatically start counting contractions and using focused breathing techniques. They are not usually necessary for the mild discomfort of early labor and will wear you out if you concentrate too hard and too soon on using them.

10. Food
Drink plenty of fluids and eat a light snack (something that is not fatty or spicy) while laboring at home. This will help to keep your energy levels up and avoid dehydration.

11. Positions
As contractions increase in intensity, try a variety of upright positions, such as standing, squatting, kneeling or rocking to lessen discomfort and facilitate labor, letting gravity work to your advantage. If your labor is predominately felt in the back, sit forward with your arms around a support person or labor on your hands and knees. Change positions frequently to improve circulation and prevent muscle fatigue.

12. Shower
Take a warm shower to help relax you and reduce muscle tension. Aim the showerhead at the lower back or wherever you are feeling your contractions the most. A warm bath or whirlpool is also okay as long as your bag of water is intact. A warm compress placed on the back, neck or abdomen also feels good on muscles that are working hard. On the other hand, in advanced labor or during pushing efforts, a cool compress will probably feel better.

13. Massage
Try a massage by your partner or birth companion. A 1997 University of Michigan study reported that women who received labor massages felt less pain and anxiety during their childbirth experience than those who were not massaged. Let the person massaging you know what feels best at different points in labor. For example, during early labor, a shoulder or neck rub may feel great, but during advanced labor, this may need to be replaced by firm pressure to the small of the back. Ultimately, you may decide you'd rather not be touched at all as labor progresses.

14. Medication

Be open to medication for relief of pain and tension if needed. Asking for and accepting medication shouldn't be viewed as a sign of failure or weakness, and it is sometimes necessary to keep a laboring woman at her best and to facilitate the birth process. While natural methods have fewer risks and side effects (these will be discussed in detail during childbirth preparation class), appropriate, timely and judicious use of medication sometimes more effectively helps reach the ultimate and most important goal of a healthy baby born to a healthy mother. A small amount of analgesia injected intravenously may dull contractions just enough to help promote relaxation so that natural strategies may be more effectively employed. An epidural (anesthetic injected into the space outside the spinal cord) may actually speed cervical dilatation by completely relaxing the pelvic muscles. The profound anesthesia provided by an epidural may also make a brief period of sleep possible and reenergize an otherwise exhausted laboring woman prior to the work of pushing the baby through the birth canal after complete dilatation is reached. If it turns out that you would benefit from medication in your labor, be glad it is available.

15. Perspective

And most importantly, throughout pregnancy and the birth process, keep your perspective. No matter how intense your childbirth experience is, it will not last forever. Most first-time labors last less than 24 hours from start to finish and of the one day of your life that childbirth involves, only a few of the hours spent are likely to be uncomfortable, especially if you have prepared adequately ahead of time. And remember each contraction brings you closer to the birth of your baby and the beginning of your new life as a parent. When all is said and done, it will probably be the most worthwhile one day of hard work you will ever engage in.

Jennifer Normoyle, MD, OB/GYN
(650) 742-2173

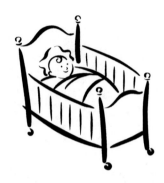

Part Seven: Choices Regarding the Moment of Birth and After

Choices Regarding the Moment of Birth and After

A new mom has several choices regarding the moments just after the birth, assuming it is a normal birth. If not, emergency measures may mean the baby is whisked from her for observation or procedures.

Otherwise, a woman can include in her birth plan how she would like these first moments to be spent. Would she like her partner to cut the cord? Would she like to bank the umbilical blood? Would she like to require that she and/or her partner are with the baby at all times?

AFTER THE BABY IS BORN

by Regula Burki, MD, FACOG

The process described here applies mostly to a normal vaginal birth, as most births take place as such. Procedures for cesarean births vary some, though changes may have to be made because of any medical problems of the mother and/or the baby that led to the need for a cesarean. Of course, medical complications that can arise at any moment even with a vaginal birth may necessitate a change from the usual routines.

FINISHING THE BIRTH

FIRST BREATH

After the baby is delivered, her nose and mouth are cleared of the amniotic fluid, blood and mucous from the birth canal. If there is meconium present (that is, the baby has had a bowel movement before or during labor and the amniotic fluid is greenish brown), not only do the nose and mouth have to be cleared but also the trachea. This may require extensive suctioning of the baby's airways, including possible intubation (insertion of a breathing tube) immediately after birth. The procedures necessary to clear the airways will depend on how thick and sticky the meconium is. Failure to clear meconium from the airways will result in severe respiratory complications, which not all newborns survive. A well equipped birthing center will have all the equipment necessary and professionals experienced in using it. After the air passages are cleared, the baby will take the first breath. Spanking is not necessary. Gently rubbing the baby's back or tapping the soles of the feet is all the stimulation required.

It is also not necessary for the baby to cry loudly. The more comfortable a healthy baby feels, the less loudly she will protest. Hearing and feeling mom is the best way to comfort a newborn.

Umbilical Cord

After the doctor or midwife is sure the baby is breathing well, the baby is usually placed on the mom's belly or chest. There is no hurry to cut the cord immediately unless a medical problem requires it. A mother can choose whom she wants to cut the cord as part of her birth plan. Unless a medical emergency arises, her wishes should be accommodated. It is a good idea, however, to remind the person delivering the baby of her preference. The birth professional may not be as current on the birth plan as the mom is!

Banking of Umbilical Cord Blood

Cord blood is the blood that remains in the umbilical cord after the baby is born. It contains special cells called stem cells; stem cells are the building blocks of the blood and immune system and potentially other body tissues. Stem cells are also found in bone marrow. Cord blood stem cells may be used instead of a bone marrow transplant to treat certain cancers, such as leukemia, and potentially may treat immune and genetic disorders. Research on the various uses of cord stem cells is ongoing.

Cord blood banking allows the preservation of these stem cells for the baby's and the family's future use if the need arises. The collection process, done after the baby is born, takes two to four minutes and is easy, painless and non-invasive. There are several companies that store babies' cord blood for a fee.

The American College of Obstetricians and Gynecologists states that "there are many questions about this technology that remain unanswered. Parents should not be sold this service without a realistic assessment of their likely return on the investment. The odds of needing a stem cell transplant are low—estimated at between one in 1,000 and one in 200,000 by age 18. Commercial cord blood banks should not represent the service they sell as 'doing everything possible' to ensure the health of children, nor should parents be made to feel guilty if they are not eager or able to invest considerable sums in such a highly speculative venture."

Apgar Score

The Apgar score was developed in 1952 as a quick way to assess how the newborn is doing overall. The score is made up of heart rate, effort to breathe, muscle tone, reflex response and color and measured at one and five minutes after birth. The maximum score is 10, 7-10 at five minutes is considered "normal."

The Apgar score is useful in evaluating how a newborn is doing right now and how well she is responding to being resuscitated, but has been found to be a poor predictor for how the baby is going to do in the long run (including on SATs) and a poor indicator of lack of oxygen during the birthing process.

Muscle tone, reflexes and color depend very much on the baby's maturity, so that premature babies get a falsely low score. Medications given to the mom during labor and certain birth defects can also produce an artificially low Apgar score.

More sophisticated methods of evaluating babies are now often being used along with the old Apgar scoring system.

Placenta

The placenta is usually expelled spontaneously within a few minutes after the birth of the baby. Sometimes the mother will be asked to give one last push to expel the placenta. Signs that the placenta is ready to be expelled are a lengthening of the umbilical cord that is still hanging out of the mom at this point and a sudden gush of blood as the placenta separates from the wall of the uterus and moves down the birth canal. If all goes well the mother will also feel her uterus turning into a hard ball that reaches about to the level of the belly button. It is perfectly safe to wait half an hour or more for the placenta to deliver, and certainly much safer than intervening too early.

Problems with the delivery of the placenta are one of the major life-threatening obstetrical complications: Postpartum hemorrhage is still the cause of death for many women in the developing world. If the placenta does not separate cleanly and completely from the wall of the uterus, the blood vessels that have been bringing blood to the baby remain wide open and pump blood out of the mom. Experienced birthing professionals have several methods to remove an incompletely separated placenta that range from uterine massage to manual removal (placing a hand inside the uterus) to medications that cause contraction of the blood vessels in the womb to surgery as a last resort. Only a well-equipped hospital has the full range of options readily available for such a complication, and maternal deaths are exceedingly rare in that setting. The delivery of the placenta is called the third stage of labor.

REPAIR OF THE EPISIOTOMY AND/OR PERINEAL TEARS
After the delivery of the placenta, any tears sustained around the vaginal opening will be repaired by placing absorbable sutures. If an episiotomy incision was made to enlarge the vaginal opening it will be repaired at this time, as well. If the mom did not have an epidural, spinal or a perineal block for the delivery, a small amount of local anesthetic is injected in the tissues before they are sutured.

TAKING CARE OF THE NEWBORN

KEEPING THE BABY WARM
It is extremely important for a newborn to be kept warm and dry. A wet newborn in an air-conditioned delivery room will rapidly lose body heat. Shivering to keep warm will increase the need for oxygen and use up precious energy stores. Placing the baby on your chest allows you to share your body heat. It also gives the mom a chance to get acquainted and even try her hand at nursing for the first time. The sensation of the baby on the nipples makes her body release hormones that induce the uterus to contract, causing the placenta to separate and preventing hemorrhage. Mother Nature planned all this very nicely. Depending on the temperature in the room the mother may want a blanket for her and the baby. Many hospitals still routinely take the baby to the nursery for a few hours for "observation" and place him in an incubator to keep warm. There is absolutely no medical reason for this as long as the baby is healthy and breathing well. The mother has been "incubating" this baby for nine month and can keep her baby warm with her own body heat and a soft blanket. All the mom has to do is say "no" to keep her baby with her! If hospital personnel insist that the baby needs to go to the nursery, the mom needs to find out why from the pediatrician. A problem big enough to require a trip to the nursery requires the presence of a baby specialist and the mom is entitled to know what is wrong.

BATHING, WEIGHING AND MEASURING
At some point, the new mom needs to relinquish her baby to be weighed, measured and bathed. Most hospitals can do these procedures right in the birthing room. Moms may have fun watching the father give his child a first bath and receive instruction on how to handle a baby. Moth-

ers should try to cooperate with the hospital staff in the timing of this. Staff will need to fill out the paperwork on the delivery before they can go home to their own families. A bath in warm water is not at all traumatic for the baby as she has been floating in warm amniotic fluid for the last few months. And all of the relatives and friends will want to know the baby's weight and length right after they have found out the baby's gender!

Around this time the baby will also get an ID bracelet and foot prints will be taken, to ward off switched identities.

Eye Care

In the first few hours after birth, usually at the time of the first bath, the baby will need to receive an antibiotic ointment in the eyes to prevent an eye infection from the bacteria she may have picked up passing through the vagina. Even normal vaginal bacteria can be harmful to the baby's eyes. Neonatal eye infections are a major cause of blindness in the third world.

Vitamins and Vaccinations

Babies are born deficient in Vitamin K, a vitamin that is essential for blood clotting. To prevent spontaneous internal hemorrhage (hemorrhagic disease of the newborn) the baby will be given a vitamin K injection. The baby will also be vaccinated against Hepatitis B.

Newborn Pictures

Another ritual that takes place after the first bath is picture taking. Commercial photographers visit the nursery and take pictures of the newborns, which are then offered to the family for sale. You can refuse to have those pictures taken and can take your own pictures.

Circumcision

Circumcision is the surgical removal of this foreskin. If it is done, it's usually done soon after birth. Although many newborn boys in the United States are circumcised, it is much less common in Europe and other parts of the world. Moslems and Jews have circumcised their male newborns for centuries.

Circumcision is a parental decision. It is not required by law or by hospital policy. According to both the American College of Obstetricians and Gynecologists (ACOG) and the American Academy of Pediatrics (AAP), there is no medical reason for a circumcision. It is purely a cultural or religious decision (and one that is currently controversial).

Taking Care of the New Mom

Watching for Hemorrhage

For the first few hours after birth it is important to make sure that the uterus remains contracted and firm to prevent excessive hemorrhage from the raw internal surface of the womb where the placenta was attached. If the woman had a very long labor, an extra large baby, or was on labor-inducing or augmenting drugs, this may require continued medications. If the mother had a spontaneous, relatively short labor, her uterus probably only needs to be massaged periodically to remind it to remain firm. She can do that herself or it can be done by the nurses who will come by to check on the new mom regularly for a few hours. One way to keep the uterus firm after birth is to have the baby suckle, as this stimulates the release of natural hormones that make the uterus contract. Mothers can also stimulate their own nipples, but that is not as much fun.

Where to Keep the Baby

In most hospitals, the mom has the option of keeping her baby with her or having the baby taken to the nursery.

Unless the mom or the baby has medical problems that require intensive care or specialized nursery care, there is absolutely no medical reason a healthy baby needs to be separated from a healthy mother. The baby is used to hearing mom's voice and body sounds from the "inside," and is reassured by hearing those same sounds after birth. The best way to calm a newborn is to place her on the left side of the mom's chest so she can be soothed by mom's heartbeat. (Later on, some babies can be "tricked" by placing an old-fashioned ticking clock next to the crib!) Birth is physically and emotionally taxing for both mom and baby. There is nothing wrong with them settling in for a good nap once the excitement of the baby's arrival into the world and all the associated ceremonies, including cleanup and family notification, are over. Before mom and baby's first nap together, however, they may want to start with breast-feeding (see next section).

On the other hand, if the mom really needs sleep and wants someone to be watching the baby, she may want to turn the baby over the competent professionals in the nursery for a few hours. After a good restoring sleep, there is plenty of time to start being a mom.

How long to stay in the hospital

The length of your hospital stay is up to you. If you choose to have an "ambulatory" delivery and leave for home only a few hours after you give birth, it is important that you have the appropriate support system lined up at home. Giving birth is an exhausting job and you cannot be expected to go home to cook and clean, do the laundry and take care of a newborn and her siblings. Your body needs time to recover. In every culture on earth there is time set aside for the new mom to recover while other women in the community take care of her and her usual duties. The more "primitive" the culture, the more "civilized" are the customs of helping out the new mother.

It is also important that the baby is evaluated regularly for the first few days of life in order to recognize problems as early as possible. You must make arrangements for home visits by a pediatric nurse if you choose to leave early.

A home health nurse will also be able to make sure you are all right and coping well with your new role. Some women will develop postpartum depression, a life threatening condition for both mother and baby, if not recognized and treated.

On the other hand, you may want to stay in the hospital as long as your insurance plan allows. This is the only time for many months when all you need to do is rest, nurse and admire your baby. Let others bring you food, clean up and do the laundry! A few years back managed care forced women and their newborns out of the hospital and pressured doctors and midwives to discharge their patients early. Women only gained the right to stay in the hospital longer than 24 hours after a tough battle that required the cooperation of medical professionals and patients as well as congressional intervention.

Staying an extra day or two also gives the nurses a chance to teach you how to take care of your baby and yourself and get you and your baby comfortable with breast-feeding.

Breast-feeding

by Jack Newman, MD, FRCPC

Breast-feeding is the *natural*, *physiologic* way of feeding infants and young children milk, and human milk is the milk made specifically for human infants. Formulas made from cows' milk or soy beans (most of them) are only superficially similar, and advertising which states otherwise is misleading. Breast-feeding should be easy and trouble free for most mothers. A good start helps to assure breast-feeding is a happy experience for both mother and baby.

The vast majority of mothers are perfectly capable of breast-feeding their babies *exclusively* for four to six months. In fact, most mothers produce *more than enough* milk. Unfortunately, outdated hospital routines based on bottle feeding *still* predominate in many health care institutions and make breast-feeding difficult, even impossible, for some mothers and babies. For breast-feeding to be well and properly established, a good early few days can be crucial. Even with a terrible start, many mothers and babies manage.

The trick to breast-feeding is getting the baby to latch on well. A baby who latches on well gets milk well. A baby who latches on poorly has difficulty getting milk, especially if the supply is low. A poor latch is similar to giving a baby a bottle with a nipple hole that is too small—the bottle is full of milk, but the baby will not get much. When a baby is latching on poorly, he may also cause the mother nipple pain. And if he does not get milk well, he will usually stay on the breast for long periods, thus aggravating the pain. Here are a few ways breast-feeding can be made easy:

1. THE BABY SHOULD BE AT THE BREAST IMMEDIATELY AFTER BIRTH.

The vast majority of newborns can be put to the breast within minutes of birth. Indeed, research has shown that, given the chance, babies only minutes old will often crawl up to the breast from the mother's abdomen and start breast-feeding all by themselves. This process may take up to an hour or longer, but the mother and baby should be given this time together to start learning about each other. Babies who "self-attach" run into far fewer breast-feeding problems. This process *does not take any effort* on the mother's part, and the excuse that it cannot be done because the mother is tired after labor is nonsense, pure and simple. Incidentally, studies have also shown that skin to skin contact between mothers and babies keeps the baby as warm as an incubator.

2. THE MOTHER AND BABY SHOULD ROOM IN TOGETHER.

There is *absolutely no medical reason* for healthy mothers and babies to be separated from each other, even for short periods. Health facilities that routinely separate mothers and babies after birth are years behind the times, and the reasons for the separation often have to do with letting parents know who is in control (the hospital) and who is not (the parents). Often bogus reasons are given for separations. One example is the baby passed meconium before birth. A baby who passes meconium and is fine a few minutes after birth will be fine and does not need to be in an incubator for several hours of "observation."

There is no evidence that mothers who are separated from their babies are better rested. On the contrary, they are more rested and less stressed when they are with their babies. Mothers and babies learn how to sleep in the same rhythm. Thus, when the baby starts waking to feed, the mother is also starting to wake up naturally. This is not as tiring for the mother as being awakened from deep sleep, as she often is if the baby is elsewhere when he wakes up. The baby shows he is ready to feed long before he starts crying. His breathing may change, for example, or he may start to stretch. The mother, being in light sleep, will awaken, her milk will start to flow, and the calm baby will be content to nurse. A baby who has been crying for some time before being tried on the breast may refuse to take the breast even if he is ravenous. Mothers and babies should be encouraged to sleep side by side in the hospital. This is a great way for a mother to rest while the baby nurses. Breastfeeding should be relaxing, *not* tiring.

3. ARTIFICIAL NIPPLES SHOULD NOT BE GIVEN TO THE BABY.
There seems to be some controversy about whether "nipple confusion" exists. Babies will take whatever method gives them a rapid flow of fluid and may refuse others that do not. Thus, in the first few days, when the mother is producing only a little milk (as nature intended), and the baby gets a bottle (as nature intended?) from which he gets rapid flow, he will tend to prefer the rapid flow method. You don't have to be a rocket scientist to figure that one out, though many health professionals, who are supposed to be helping you, don't seem to be able to manage it. Nipple confusion includes not just the baby refusing the breast, but also the baby not taking the breast as well as he could and thus not getting milk well and/or the mother getting sore nipples. Just because a baby will "take both" does not mean that the bottle is not having a negative effect. Since there are now alternatives available if the baby needs to be supplemented, why use an artificial nipple?

4. NO RESTRICTION SHOULD BE PLACED ON THE LENGTH OR FREQUENCY OF BREAST-FEEDINGS.
A baby who drinks well will not be on the breast for hours at a time. Thus, if he is, it is usually because he is not latching on well and not getting the milk that is available. Get help to fix the baby's latch and use

compression to get the baby more milk. This, *not* a pacifier, *not* a bottle, *not* taking the baby to the nursery, will help.

5. SUPPLEMENTS OF WATER, SUGAR WATER, OR FORMULA ARE RARELY NEEDED.

Most supplements could be avoided by getting the baby to take the breast properly and get the milk that is available. If you are being told you need to supplement without someone having observed you breastfeeding, ask for someone to help who knows what they are doing. There *are* rare indications for supplementation, but usually supplements are suggested for the convenience of the hospital staff. If supplements are required, they should be given by lactation aid—not cup, finger feeding, syringe or bottle. The best supplement is your own colostrum. It can be mixed with sugar water if you are not able to express much at first. Formula is hardly ever necessary in the first few days.

6. A PROPER LATCH IS CRUCIAL TO SUCCESS.

This is the key to successful breast-feeding. Unfortunately, too many mothers are being "helped" by people who don't know what a proper latch is. If you are being told your two day old's latch is good despite your having very sore nipples, be skeptical and ask for help from someone who knows.

Before you leave the hospital, you should be shown that your baby is latched on properly, that he is actually getting milk from the breast, and that you know how to tell he is getting milk from the breast (open—*pause*—close, type of suck). If you and the baby are leaving hospital *not* knowing this, get help quickly.

7. FREE FORMULA SAMPLES AND FORMULA LITERATURE ARE NOT GIFTS.

There is only one purpose for these "gifts" and that is to get you to use formula. It is very effective, and very unethical, marketing. If you get any from a health professional, you should be wondering about his/her knowledge of breast-feeding and his/her commitment to breast-feeding. "But I need formula because the baby is not getting enough!" Maybe, but more likely, you weren't given *good* help, and the baby is simply not getting your milk well. Get good help. Formula samples are not help.

Under some circumstances, it may be impossible to start breast-feeding early. However, most medical reasons (maternal medication, for example) are *not* true reasons for stopping or delaying breast-feeding, and you are getting *mis*information. Get good help. Premature babies can start breast-feeding *much, much* earlier than they do in many health facilities. In fact, studies are now quite definite that it is *easier* for a premature baby to breast-feed than to bottle feed. Unfortunately, too many health professionals dealing with premature babies do not seem to be aware of this.

Some Breast-feeding Myths

1. MANY WOMEN DO NOT PRODUCE ENOUGH MILK.

<u>Not true</u>! The vast majority of women produce *more than enough* milk. Indeed, an *overabundance of milk* is common. Most babies who gain weight too slowly, or lose weight, do so not because the mother does not have enough milk, but because the baby does not get the milk that the mother has. The usual reason that the baby does not get the milk that is available is that he is poorly latched onto the breast. This is why it is so important that the mother be shown, on the first day, how to latch a baby on properly by someone who knows what they are doing.

2. IT IS NORMAL FOR BREAST-FEEDING TO HURT.

<u>Not true</u>! Though some tenderness during the first few days is relatively common, this should be a temporary situation which lasts only a few days, and should never be so bad that the mother dreads nursing. Any pain that is more than mild is abnormal and is almost always due to the baby latching on poorly. Any nipple pain that is not getting better by day three or four or lasts beyond five or six days should not be ignored. A new onset of pain when things have been going well for a while may be due to a yeast infection of the nipples. Limiting feeding time does not prevent soreness.

3. THERE IS NO (NOT ENOUGH) MILK DURING THE FIRST THREE OR FOUR DAYS AFTER BIRTH.

<u>Not true</u>! It often seems like that because the baby is not latched on properly and therefore is unable to get the milk. Once the mother's milk is abundant, a baby can latch on poorly and still may get plenty of milk. However, during the first few days, the baby who is latched on poorly cannot get milk. This accounts for "but he's been on the breast for two hours and is still hungry when I take him off." By not latching on well, the baby is unable to get the mother's first milk, called colostrum. Anyone who suggests you pump your milk to know how much colostrum there is does not understand breast-feeding and should be politely ignored.

4. A BABY SHOULD BE ON THE BREAST 20 MINUTES ON EACH SIDE.

Not true! However, a distinction needs to be made between "being on the breast" and "*breast-feeding.*" If a baby is *actually drinking* for most of 15-20 minutes on the first side, he may not want to take the second side at all. If he drinks only a minute on the first side and then nibbles or sleeps and does the same on the other, no amount of time will be enough. The baby will breast-feed better and longer *if he is latched on properly.* He can also be helped to breast-feed longer if the mother compresses the breast to keep the flow of milk going once he no longer swallows on his own. Thus it is obvious that the rule of thumb that "the baby gets 90% of the milk in the breast in the first 10 minutes" is equally hopelessly wrong.

5. A BREAST-FEEDING BABY NEEDS EXTRA WATER IN HOT WEATHER.

Not true! Breastmilk contains all the water a baby needs.

6. BREAST-FEEDING BABIES NEED EXTRA VITAMIN D.

Not true! Except in extraordinary circumstances (for example, if the mother herself was vitamin D deficient during the pregnancy). The baby stores vitamin D during the pregnancy and a little outside exposure, on a regular basis, gives the baby all the vitamin D he needs.

7. A MOTHER SHOULD WASH HER NIPPLES BEFORE FEEDING THE BABY.

Not True! Formula feeding requires careful attention to cleanliness because formula not only does not protect the baby against infection, but also is a good breeding ground for bacteria and can be easily contaminated. On the other hand, breast milk protects the baby against infection. Washing nipples before each feeding makes breast-feeding unnecessarily complicated and washes away protective oils from the nipple.

8. PUMPING IS A GOOD WAY OF KNOWING HOW MUCH MILK THE MOTHER HAS.

Not true! How much milk can be pumped depends on many factors, including the mother's stress level. The baby who nurses well can get much more milk than his mother can pump. Pumping only tells you how much you can pump.

9. BREAST MILK DOES NOT CONTAIN ENOUGH IRON FOR THE BABY'S NEEDS.

<u>Not true</u>! Breastmilk contains just enough iron for the baby's needs. If the baby is full term, he will get enough iron from breastmilk to last him at least the first six months. Formulas contain *too much* iron, but this quantity may be necessary to *ensure the baby absorbs enough* to prevent iron deficiency. The iron in formula is *poorly* absorbed, and most of it, the baby poops out. Generally, there is no need to add other foods to breastmilk before about six months of age.

10. IT IS EASIER TO BOTTLE FEED THAN TO BREAST-FEED.

<u>Not true</u>! Or this should not be true. However, breast-feeding is made difficult because women often do not receive the help they should to get started properly. A poor start can indeed make breast-feeding difficult. But a poor start can also be overcome. Breast-feeding is often more difficult at first due to a poor start, but usually becomes easier later.

11. BREAST-FEEDING TIES THE MOTHER DOWN.

<u>Not true</u>! But it depends how you look at it. A baby can be nursed anywhere, anytime, and thus breast-feeding is *liberating* for the mother. No need to drag around bottles or formula. No need to worry about where to warm up the milk. No need to worry about sterility. No need to worry about how your baby is because he is with you.

12. THERE IS NO WAY TO KNOW HOW MUCH BREAST MILK THE BABY IS GETTING.

<u>Not true</u>! There is no easy way to measure how much the baby is getting, but this does not mean that you cannot know if the baby is getting enough. The best way to know is that the baby actually drinks at the breast for several minutes at each feeding (open—*pause*—close type of suck). ...

13. MODERN FORMULAS ARE ALMOST THE SAME AS BREASTMILK.

<u>Not true</u>! The same claim was made in 1900 and earlier. Modern formulas are only superficially similar to breastmilk. Every correction of a *deficiency* in formulas is advertised as an advance. Fundamentally they are inexact copies based on outdated and *incomplete* knowledge of what breastmilk is. Formulas contain no antibodies, no living cells, no enzymes, no hormones. They contain much more aluminum, manganese, cadmium and iron than breastmilk. They contain significantly more

protein than breastmilk. The proteins and fats are fundamentally different from those in breastmilk. Formulas do not vary from the beginning of the feed to the end of the feed, or from day one to day seven to day 30, or from woman to woman, or from baby to baby.... Your breastmilk is made as required to suit *your* baby. Formulas are made to suit every baby and thus *no* baby. Formulas succeed only at making babies grow well, usually, but there is more to breast-feeding than getting the baby to grow quickly.

14. IF THE MOTHER HAS AN INFECTION, SHE SHOULD STOP BREAST-FEEDING.
Not true! With very, very few exceptions, the baby will be protected by the mother continuing to breast-feed. By the time the mother has a fever (or cough, vomiting, diarrhea, rash, etc.) she has already given the baby the infection, since she has been infectious for several days before she even knew she was sick. The baby's best protection against getting the infection is for the mother to continue breast-feeding. If the baby does get sick, he will be less sick if the mother continues breast-feeding. Besides, maybe it was the baby who gave the infection to the mother, but the baby did not show signs of illness because he was breast-feeding. Also, breast infections, including breast abscess, though painful, are not reasons to stop breast-feeding. Indeed, the infection is likely to settle more quickly if the mother continues breast-feeding on the affected side.

15. IF THE BABY HAS DIARRHEA OR VOMITING, THE MOTHER SHOULD STOP BREAST-FEEDING.
Not true! The best medicine for a baby's gut infection is breast-feeding. Stop other foods for a short time, but continue breast-feeding. Breastmilk is the *only* fluid your baby requires when he has diarrhea and/or vomiting, except under exceptional circumstances. The push to use "oral rehydrating solutions" is mainly a push by the formula (and oral rehydrating solution) manufacturers to make even more money. The baby is comforted by the breast-feeding, and the mother is comforted by the baby's breast-feeding.

16. IF THE MOTHER IS TAKING MEDICINE, SHE SHOULD NOT BREAST-FEED.
Not true! There are very, very few medicines that a mother cannot take safely while breast-feeding. A very small amount of most medicines appears in the milk, but usually in such small quantities that there is no

concern. If a medicine is truly of concern, there are usually equally effective alternative medicines that are safe. The loss of benefit of breast-feeding for both the mother and the baby *must be taken into account* when weighing if breast-feeding should be continued.

Jack Newman graduated from the University of Toronto Medical School as a pediatrician in 1970. He started the first hospital-based breast-feeding clinic in Canada in 1984 at Toronto's Hospital for Sick Children. He has been a consultant with UNICEF for the Baby Friendly Hospital Initiative in Africa and has published articles on the subject of breast-feeding in Scientific American and several medical journals. Dr. Newman has practised as a physician in Canada, New Zealand, and South Africa. Dr. Newman's book on breast-feeding is called The Ultimate Breast-feeding Book of Answers (published in the U.S. by Prima Publishing, August 2000) or Dr. Jack Newman's Guide to Breast-feeding (published in Canada by HarperCollins, February 2000).

Reprinted with the permission of Dr. Newman.

WHERE TO GET HELP FOR BREAST-FEEDING
from La Leche League International

LA LECHE LEAGUE—A LOVING WAY OF LIFE

Founded in 1956 by seven women who had learned about successful breast-feeding while nursing their own babies, La Leche League is the only organization with the sole purpose of helping breast-feeding mothers.

Now 8,000 leaders and 3,000 local groups strong in the United States alone, La Leche League has groups that meet regularly in communities worldwide to share breast-feeding information and mothering experience. Each year, an estimated 750,000 American mothers call La Leche League with questions and concerns. Telephone counseling is available 24 hours a day, along with access to an extensive library of breast-feeding literature.

When a woman joins La Leche League, she participates in a mother-to-mother helping network, a priceless resource for breast-feeding and parenting help, support, knowledge, and inspiration.

Breast-feeding is a wonderfully simple and natural process, but mothers do need support and information on such topics as the correct positioning of the baby at the breast, working and breast-feeding, avoiding problems, and overcoming any difficulties that may occur. Questions also arise: Is my baby getting enough to eat? How can I tell? Why is my baby fussing? What can the father do to participate in caring for the baby? When should my baby wean? And so forth. Feel free to call your local La Leche League Leader with your questions.

HOW TO FIND A LA LECHE LEAGUE LEADER NEAR YOU

- Contact at www.lalecheleague.org
- Look in your local telephone directory. Many La Leche League groups have listings in the white or yellow pages. Some are also listed in the free "blue" pages for nonprofit organizations. If there is no listing under "La Leche League," look under headings labeled "breast-feeding" or "lactation." In some places, La Leche League will be listed under "community resources" or "women's health."
- Call your pediatrician or health clinic. They often have a file of La Leche League Leader's names. Your local library may also have a listing.
- If there is no online resource near you and you can't find us locally, pick up your telephone and dial 1-800-LALECHE (U.S.) or (847) 519-7730. You will be referred through a recording to a La Leche League Leader near you.

Information reprinted with permission of La Leche League International.

ADDITIONAL BREAST-FEEDING SUPPORT

INTERNATIONAL LACTATION CONSULTANT ASSOCIATION

The ILCA has listings of certified lactation consultants in your area. You want to look for the initials IBCLC. They stand for International Board-certified Lactation Consultant, and mean that the lactation consultant has met a required number of counseling hours and passed a test on various breast-feeding topics and situations. To locate an IBCLC, contact the ILCA. You will be referred to three IBCLCs in your area.
ILCA
1500 Sunday Drive, Suite 102
Raleigh, NC 27607
phone: 919-861-5577
fax: 919-787-4916
website: www.ilca.org, email: info@ilca.org

Women's, Infants' and Children's Program (WIC)

WIC provides nutritional counseling, food supplements and breast-feeding support for pregnant and lactating women and their young children. Most WIC services require that you meet low-income guidelines. Many WIC offices have lactation consultants or specially trained health care personnel available to assist mothers with breast-feeding. You can find WIC in your local phone book. Call to find out what services they have available.

Bedrest
Questions to Ask Your Doctor or Midwife

1. How long do I need to spend on bedrest?
2. How should I change my general activity level?
3. Can I work outside the home? Can I work at home?
4. How much walking can I do?
5. How much standing can I do?
6. Can I drive on a daily basis?
7. Can I drive to doctor/midwife appointments?
8. Can I do any household chores?
9. What about childcare? Do I need to get help?
10. Can I lift anything? Are there any weight restrictions?
11. Are there any exercises I can do while on bedrest?
12. What level of sexual activity can I have?
13. Can I move around the house during the day?
14. What position should I rest in?
15. Can I take a shower/bath?
16. Can I get up to use the toilet?
17. Are there any symptoms or signs that I should pay special attention to?

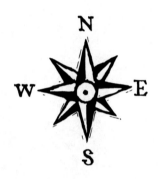

Part Eight: Birth Customs Around the World

Birth Around the World

In the society in which we live, pregnancy and birth are viewed as medical conditions with many associated risks. Women and their partners consult with medical personnel who counsel them on the expectations and risks that are involved. Most expectant parents plan to have their baby in a hospital surrounded by a trained medical staff and technical equipment. Birth has not always been viewed like this, and in many cultures around the world, it is still not. By looking to other cultures, we can enrich our own birth culture by designing births that care for the soul as well as the physical needs of the mother and baby.

Pregnancy

In many third world cultures, human pregnancy is believed to be the force that makes the crops grow and animals bear young. There is an interconnection between human fertility and the productivity of nature. They are both part of a greater organic whole. The fertility of the land and the animals, and the spoils of hunting depend on human fertility. When women in the village are pregnant, all will be well with the harvest and the food supply.

How pregnancy is announced is also very different around the world. In some cultures, it is hidden until the very end because disclosing it was considered to bring bad luck. In order to have a healthy baby in rural Greece and Ireland, this was the case until very recently. Vietnamese women avoid mentioning their due dates and Hmong women are uncomfortable mentioning the expected date of birth when completing paperwork in medical clinics. In the Jewish tradition, women often kept a pregnancy secret, and many Ashkenazi Jews still feel happier doing so. Sephardic Jews in the Ottoman Empire were an exception. They celebrated with a pregnancy rite, *Kortadura de Fashadura*, "the cutting of the swaddling bands." Women gathered to make the first swaddling cloth and the pregnant woman threw sugared almonds onto the swaddling cloth to represent the sweet life that she wished for her baby. In our own culture, many women wait until three or four months have passed and there is less risk of miscarriage before announcing their pregnancy.

In Fiji, pregnancy is announced immediately. The pregnancy becomes the responsibility of the entire community with everyone offering advice and comments. Traditionally among the Maori in New Zealand a female choir sings to the baby and the expectant mother about the progress of her pregnancy. If things are not going well or they detect signs that the baby is not developing normally they sing about this, too, in the *marae*, the great wooden temple in which the communal life of the people is conducted and which represents the spirit of the tribe. Each pregnancy links women together in shared pleasure or concern.

In all cultures, quickening (the first feeling of life) is recognized as an important transition in the process of becoming a mother. In Bulgaria, it is the point at which a woman would bake bread and take it as an offering to the church, letting everyone know that she was pregnant. Historically in Europe, women often delayed telling anyone else about a pregnancy before they felt quickening. "Quick" is old English for "alive," as in the phrase "the quick and the dead." In non-technological cultures, women get to know their unborn babies through awareness of their movements. In our own culture, the ultrasound is often the first way we come to know our future child. Once again, we must rely on the knowledge and training of medical personnel before this is possible.

Today many pregnant women believe that they can communicate with the baby inside them and affect the baby's character in a positive way. Japanese parenting magazines are packed with articles about how talking to the baby, playing music, massaging the uterus and touching the different parts of the baby can raise a baby's IQ level and might even produce a genius. This idea is also prevalent in our own culture. There is one particular American approach to prenatal education, for example, called "The University of the Womb."

THE PROGRESSION OF PREGNANCY

Pregnancy is divided into trimesters only in countries that follow the medical model of pregnancy. Cultural perceptions of time in pregnancy, relating to the growth of the baby and the physical state of the mother, shape an image of pregnancy that is usually not anchored to specific states or stages. It is seen as an organic whole with its own rhythms, which are independent of the calendar or medical charts.

In some cultures, however, pregnancy ceremonies are linked to the religious calendar. In Japan, for example, the Day of the Dog in the fifth month of pregnancy, according to the Shinto religious calendar, is associated with the rite that celebrates the pregnancy and guards the baby against harm. The Dog, one of the twelve animals of the zodiac that form the ancient oriental calendar, is a messenger from the gods and chases evil spirits away. It is an auspicious time for the presentation of the expectant mother at the temple and for the donning of the *hara-obi*—the sash that protects her baby, ensures that it stays "down" and keeps it "warm." She goes to the Shinto temple with her mother-in-law and often with both prospective grandmothers to get the *obi* from the priest and have it blessed. The women pray together at the shrine.

PREGNANCY RITES AROUND THE WORLD

In Bali, parents believe that they help their baby grow strong and healthy when they conduct the ceremony of *pegedong-gedoonga* ("building") around the sixth month of pregnancy. The actual time is not dependent on the calendar, but is indicated when the mother starts to crave sour foods, as it is considered that the baby then has full human form. This private prayer ceremony takes place in the bathing area of the household compound. From that point on, the four spirit brothers or sisters, the *kanda empot*, protect and nourish the fetus. These spirits are also born with the baby and continue to watch over the child.

In India, Bemata is the goddess of the life force that nurtures the unborn child, just as she nurtures all plants with their roots in the earth. She lives beneath the earth and throws the baby into the woman's uterus. The *dai*, a midwife, is the "earth mother" and works with Bemata to see that the baby is born safely. In the seventh month of pregnancy, the expectant mother performs a rite in which she worships a tree. She does this to give thanks to the spirit that lives in the tree and protects her body by offering her sari blouse and hanging it on a branch.

Among the Navajo Hosooji in North America, the Blessing Way ceremony for "Long-Life Empowering" is enacted during the pregnancy. It lasts nine days and involves the use of herbs, chanting and an all-night rite called "No-Sleep." Following this, as the sun rises, the pregnant woman goes to the door and breathes deeply, visualizing "the perfect world seen by the Holy People at the dawn of the Fifth World— the world of beauty, thought, and knowledge." A Blessing Way chanter says, "You inhale the dawn four times and give a prayer to yourself, the dawn and everything that exists. Everything is made holy again."

A similar sunrise ceremony, including deep breathing and prayer, is an important pregnancy rite in South Africa among the Zulu. Each morning the woman goes outside her hut and breathes deeply to empty herself of evil.

PREPARATION FOR BIRTH

In most cultures, it is believed that a woman can also help prepare for safe and easy birth by the way she behaves in pregnancy. In Jamaica, for example, she must avoid stepping over a donkey's tethering rope, lest the umbilical cord becomes tightly drawn around the baby's neck. In Sicily, a pregnant woman is careful not to twist her necklace or to wear a tight scarf for the same reason. The Navajo believe that to avoid knots in the cord, a pregnant woman must not sit with crossed legs.

Objects that are crossed or knotted and positions of the body that represent tightness or closure are believed to affect the way a woman's body works in labor, too, so that her cervix may not open easily. As she reaches the time when her baby is due, she may be advised to undo knots in her clothing and avoid tying anything up. The Sicilian expectant mother is told to sit with her knees well apart and never to cross her legs. Everything should be open and loose. It is possible that this concentration of thinking has a strong psychosomatic effect, and that it is one way of psychological preparation for birth.

In some cultures, women protect their pregnancies with amulets, charms and prayers. Christians pray to Saint Anne, Saint Gerard and the Virgin Mary. In many other religions, fertility goddesses watch over women during pregnancy and birth. The expectant woman may wear a pregnancy sash or belt to protect the baby. Navajo women wear a bright red sash for this purpose. In peasant Mexico, the sash, the *muneco*, is also used by the visiting midwife to measure fundal height. The pregnancy sash often has a sacred quality. The "girdle of Mary," worn by Englishwomen in the Middle Ages, was handed down through mothers and daughters in the family, as was the ancient Greek girdle.

In England, girdles were often kept in convents and loaned to pregnant women in childbirth, too. This is how the red silk Our Lady's girdle of Bruton was used. The Jewish girdles were sometimes embroidered and later used for binding the Torah, the book of Judaic law.

PRENATAL CARE

A common part of prenatal care in many cultures is massage. An older woman in the family—the mother or mother-in-law or the village midwife—regularly massages the woman's back, abdomen, arms, and legs using whatever vegetable oil is available locally. In Fiji and Indonesia, it is coconut oil. In Mediterranean countries, it is olive oil. Home visits by the midwife often include abdominal palpitation at the same time as massage while the two women talk together about how the expectant mother is feeling and how the pregnancy is progressing.

Among Mayans in Guatemala, the midwife is formally requested to visit the pregnant woman with a gift of food and money to buy candles and incense for St. Anne and other saints. Midwives in South American cultures listen to the heartbeat directly with an ear against the abdomen. The expectant mother may bathe her perineum in an infusion of avocado leaves and salt to make the tissues strong, soft and flexible. In many cultures, she also massages her perineum. In Jamaica, the oil of the wild castor oil plant and the juicy pulp of toona leaves are used.

The belief is common in most cultures that a woman's body should be powerful and lithe for birth. To give birth with ease, a woman should remain physically active during pregnancy, especially in the last weeks. If an expectant mother lies around, it is thought that her labor will be more difficult. Navajo women are advised to walk a lot to help the circulation and keep the baby small enough to pass through the pelvis without difficulty.

After birth in traditional societies, respite from physical labor is linked with rites of postpartum segregation and nurturing by other women; a new mother is assured a break from work and some kind of sanctuary for a short time after giving birth. Rather than wanting to "get back to normal" as soon as possible after birth, now the norm in industrialized cultures, an Asian woman who has just had a baby expects to be cared for and rest while others do the work. This conflicts with the attitude of nurses who want to get the new mother on her feet, caring for the baby herself and taking responsibility in the early days following the birth.

In most countries throughout history, only socially privileged women had other women to do their regular work for them. The concept of prenatal exercises developed because women who were comfortably off often became physically inactive. Their muscles were untoned, circulation sluggish and bodies stiff because they no longer had to scrub floors and till the land, and because, in the 20th century, they acquired labor-saving machines that required less effort and could do at least some household tasks for them.

Throughout the third world, women squat and kneel in positions in which the pelvis is at its widest and, in their work, make movements in which the pelvis rocks, tilts and rotates in a smooth and steady rhythm. These movements, which are the basis of exercises practiced in pregnancy classes in northern industrialized cultures, are elements in the daily work of rural women in South America, the Pacific Islands, Africa and the Indian subcontinent. They are also components of the dances that universally are part of women's culture. The same movements are used when a woman is in labor, and women helpers encourage her by rocking and circling their own pelvises in the same rhythm. Bedouin Arab girls are taught these movements formally after they have had their first period, both for sex and for childbirth. What we know as belly dancing is essentially a fertility dance in which women celebrate the power to give life.

Historically in Europe, there seems to have been no specific exercises with which to prepare for birth, though what is now known as folk dance was a regular form of celebration in every rural community.

Birth

In most cultures, the midwife is not merely a birth attendant, she also has a spiritual quality and role. Traditional midwives in the Philippines, *hilots*, combine practical and supernatural skills guided by the spirits of ancestors who were "gifted" in the same way. A World Health Organization (WHO) report states that they are revered in their communities. They know how to dispose of the placenta so that evil spirits cannot find it; and since "the Gate of Heaven" is open for forty-four days after childbirth, they attend the mother throughout this time massaging and binding her abdomen, as well as helping with the housework and other children.

Similarly, midwives in Malaysia can deal with evil spirits and prevent them from attacking the mother and baby. The *bidan* understand the rites that must be enacted to purify the woman and make her less vulnerable to these spirits, the positions she should adopt to avoid them, and how to make the house safe with the leaves of prickly *pandanus* and charms to bar their way.

Sometimes midwives use the image of a flower, one that opens as the cervix dilates, to help a woman focus on the opening of her body. It is a common practice in southern India, Malaysia and in rural parts of Mediterranean countries, such as southern Italy and Greece. The birth flower is the rose of Jericho. Apparently dry and shriveled, it is placed beside the mother and gradually spreads wide all its petals in the heat of the birth room. It is an intense visual image. In the Christian tradition, the same flower is known in Italy as "the rose of Mary." In Greece, it is "the hand of the Mother of God."

Prayer is one way of creating and sustaining harmony with spiritual forces. In Hawaii, the midwife was called Kahuna Pale Keiki and was also a priest. After praying to the Goddess of Childbirth, she could take away the mother's pain and transfer it from her to anyone she chose. In many cultures, there are special birth prayers and invocations. In both the Jewish and Muslim faith, for example, there are birth prayers to be recited by the father while his wife labors, and others to celebrate the baby's birth.

The ways birthing women are cared for can be very different from the quiet, intimate birth scenes that we have come to associate with sensitive, skilled midwifery in birth centers and at home births today. Very large female groups may gather. The result is a noisy bustle of activity. Anthropologists who have been present at a birth often sound quite shocked by the crowds, the banter and gossip in the birth room. These women share a sense of purpose. The practical work of birth is the central reason for their coming together. Yet childbirth is, above all, an opportunity for asserting female solidarity and reinforcing bonds.

Throughout Europe in medieval times, a woman called on friends and neighbors to attend her in childbirth and care for her in the days afterwards. If need be, some of them stayed for weeks doing the cooking; washing; looking after the other children; seeing that the necessary tasks in the dairy, herb-garden or small holding were carried out; and, in a peasant household, milking the cow and feeding the pigs and chickens. These women were known as god-sibs—literally "sisters in God." Birth took place within female territory from which men were excluded. They left the house and women took over. The word "God-sib" gradually changed in male language to "gossip."

In Egypt today, the group helping the birthing woman includes her mother, her husband's mother, her husband's sisters, her own sisters, paternal aunts and perhaps a neighbor, as well as a midwife. They hold her in their arms or support her back in a squatting, kneeling or sitting position, depending on how she is most comfortable at the time and what the midwife advises.

The Seri are a small tribe who live in one of the driest, poorest areas of Mexico. Most women are now transported to hospitals to have their babies, but there is a strong tradition of woman-to-woman help. The Seri mother decides whom she wants with her at the birth. They are usually close relatives. They help her position herself for labor and birth and one of them is ready to catch the baby when it is born. These women prepare special teas to help the birth, and after the baby is delivered, they bind a long piece of cloth tightly around the mother's fundus to aid the expulsion of the placenta, massage her abdomen, and give her other special teas. Once the placenta is delivered, they wrap hot stones in a cloth or heat bundles of twigs and place them against her body to ease after-pains. The baby is washed and dressed, and one of the women offers sweetened water from a clam shell and rests the baby in the mother's arms. They also have the task of keeping a ritual fire burning in the home for four days after the birth in order to "fire" the baby, much as a clay pot is fired in a kiln. Since neither parent is supposed to work for at least four days after the birth, these women take on the household tasks, though in practice, the father usually has to get back to the fields and the mother does a little light washing.

Today, most Inuit women in northern Canada are not allowed to give birth in their own communities. They are transported to hospitals hundreds of miles away. Previously, they gave birth with the help of their mothers and mothers-in-law together with other female family members and neighbors and often their husbands as well. There were usually at least three helping women present, and the father was much more actively involved than is the case today. Before they lived in settlements, women gave birth in igloos, tents, and temporary log cabins, sometimes in the open, in boats and even on moving sledges (heavy sleds). Knowledge about birth was shared among all those who helped, and in many camps, there was no particular individual with specialized training. Every woman was educated to assist.

Japan also has a strong tradition of woman-to-woman help in childbirth. Historically, besides the midwife, the *samba*, both grandmothers, often assisted, together with other women from the neighborhood. Still today, a woman may go to her mother's house a month before the birth and, although she usually has a hospital delivery, is cared for by her mother and female relatives.

Dutch birth culture has always been women-centered, but usually has involved the father as well. For many Dutch women, birth remains a domestic process and many go through the whole of their pregnancy and birth without seeing a doctor. Thirty percent of births still take place at home. The state also provides women helpers who come into the home, supplementing or taking the place of the care given by female family members. This training was first established at the turn of the century because, with rapid urbanization, couples often moved to towns where they had no other family. In 1926, the government started to sponsor the scheme nationally and it remains an important part of maternity care. The helping woman, or *kraamverzorgende*, assists during the birth, cares for the mother and baby afterwards, and does the housekeeping and cooking.

There is now a developing awareness in modern hospitals of the value of woman-to-woman support through labor. It is not only that mothers are happier when they have another woman with them, but also that birth is easier and safer. Female companionship is the one element in care that has been shown to be the most effective in keeping birth normal. The term often used is doula, first suggested by the anthropologist Dana Raphael. Penny Simkin began to train doulas—

women who give time to support other women in childbirth, not as midwives, but as sisters sharing the experience—at the Seattle Midwifery School in 1988 because her research on the long-term impact of women's first birth experiences revealed that women remember their births vividly, and often poignantly, even twenty years later. Their level of satisfaction is strongly associated not with the length of labor, with complications, or whether they had drugs for pain relief, but with the way they were treated by those caring for them. In 1992, she started Doulas of North America, and now over 3,000 doulas are being trained annually. (See the section "All About Doulas" for more information.)

THE BIRTH PLACE

When women design their own birth space, it is very different from the usual hospital delivery room with a large clock and a bed or central delivery table. They choose a pool, candles, soft indirect lighting, pictures that have special meaning for them, comfortable floor cushions and perhaps a rocking chair and a birth stool. When they are free to move, they often give birth in a secluded corner of the room. Bianca Lepori is an Italian architect who has studied the spontaneous movements women make in labor and how, given an intimate space, they use various parts of it to walk, crouch, stand or be on all fours. She designs birth rooms that follow these movements, rather than imposing an expectation that the woman will lie down on the bed or give birth in the center of the room. She incorporates into her designs a curved birth pool and lighting that can be dimmed, and which is often mysterious and subtle. Another Italian architect, Fanny Di Cara, imagines an open-air garden or courtyard space for birth that includes trees, flowers, flowing water and a log fire.

The ways that a woman is allowed to position herself for labor and delivery vary from culture to culture. However, women all over the world spontaneously squat, kneel, stand or lean forward to give birth. Birth stools and chairs evolved from lap-sitting and squatting positions. While births stools and chairs have improved over time, a bean bag on the floor or a couple's double bed remain the most comfortable places to give birth.

Water also has become more important in birthing. While it has always been a part of birth, water birth—immersion in a birth pool—is a modern invention. Dr. Michel Odent first offered women the chance of laboring in water at his clinic in Pithiviers. He did not plan for them to give birth in water—this happened because the labor progressed so quickly that there was no time to get the woman out! Now one can rent a birth pool. (See the section "Water Birth" for more information.)

THE IMPORTANCE OF TOUCH

A vital element in both the art and the science of midwifery is the skill of the midwife's hands. Together with her eyes and ears, her hands are her most valuable tool. But they are more than a tool. She communicates with them. She receives information through the sensitivity of her touch and gives comfort, confidence and courage by touch. A good midwife knows exactly how and when to touch, just as she knows when to be hands off. Unfortunately, in the medical model of childbirth, touch is most often used solely for diagnostic purposes.

We have seen already that the traditional Japanese word for midwife is *samba*, "the elderly woman who massages." The heart of traditional Japanese midwifery lies in the use of touch to reposition the baby, help the woman relax and so let her body work, and to give comfort. A Mexican *partera* explained that an important part of her work was touching "as soft as I can." Yet it is not only the *partera* who touches. The *tendera*, another woman who nurtures the mother during childbirth, also holds and touches. While the *tendera* supports her from behind, the *partera* sits in front of her.

Almost everywhere in the world, birth is followed by massage of the mother and the baby and the application of heat. In India, the *dai* massages the sides of the mother's uterus to ensure that all "dark blood" and clots (*gandagi*) flow back to the earth from whence they came. The rich blood that nurtured the baby within the uterus is personified as the Goddess Bemata, meaning "mother's love." Once the child is born, she comes down seeking the baby she has lost; this is a dangerous phase of birth. Good blood has become "bad blood." The uterus must be encouraged to contract and involute, and bleeding is welcomed as a sign that this is happening. To retain clots and polluting darkblood inside the uterus is to risk death. Massage enables blood to flow freely and the woman's open body to become closed.

The placenta is considered the sibling or the "mother" of the child. It is invariably handled with respect and often reverence, for it is the baby's tree of life, and it is ritually buried or burned. When a woman dies after childbirth, it is because this has not happened and the placenta, which is the "other mother," has "gone up and killed her."

In traditional cultures, there is a strong focus on the physical elements of mothering in the first postpartum weeks, on prolonged skin contact between mother and baby, oiling and massage, and firm binding with strips of cloth. These are primarily tactile experiences; to them are added the psychophysiological effects of heat, fire and steam bathing. There may be something that we can learn from traditional patterns of nurturing the new mother and baby, and from the tactile experiences that could facilitate and enrich the postpartum experience for women today.

In researching preparation for birth, birth itself and the postpartum period in other times and cultures, it becomes evident that our own birth culture is lacking. We must all strive to take what we can and improve the way that we approach birth for the good of each mother, baby and "new family" being created.

This entire section was made possible by the research and dedication of Sheila Kitzinger. Sheila is an anthropologist of birth and a wonderful resource for information on women's experiences of pregnancy and motherhood. Her books include The Experience of Childbirth and Pregnancy and Childbirth. Her latest book is Rediscovering Birth. For more information, visit her web site at www.sheilakitzinger.com.

Part Nine: Designing Your Birth Plan

Designing Your Birth Plan

Before you begin designing your birth plan, it may be interesting to see what other moms have desired.

Birth Plan Statistics

The following statistics are based on birth plans compiled on amazingpregnancy.com, where the user has elected to save the birth plan:

Location of Birth
Where will the birth take place
- Hospital — 85%
- Birth Center — 4%
- Home Birth — 1%
- Other location — 10%

Special Notes
- I have tested positive for Group B Strep. — 4%
- My blood type is rhesus negative. — 13%
- I have gestational diabetes. — 2%
- I am a diabetic. — 1%
- My hearing is impaired. — 1%
- My vision is impaired. — 5%

General Comments
- I would like all staff to discuss all procedures with my partner/coach and me before they are performed. — 92%
- I would like to be able to vocalize during labor and birth without criticism or comment. — 76%
- I would like permission to see my chart and the baby's chart. — 84%

Environment
- I would like the room to be quiet during labor. — 47%
- I would like it if nonessential personnel, including interns and students were not present. — 66%
- I would like a private birthing room. — 73%
- I would like my partner to be present at all times. — 94%
- I would like to wear my own choice of clothes. — 44%

I would like a private phone to be available.	64%
I would like my supporters to be able to take photographs of the labor and delivery.	65%
I would like my supporters to be able to video the labor and delivery.	43%
I would like to listen to my choice of music.	63%
I would like the lights to be dimmed.	49%
I would like to use aromatherapy during labor.	17%
I would like to have massages during labor.	55%
I would like people to respect my privacy by knocking before entering the room.	77%

During The Labor

I would like vaginal exams to be kept to a minimum.	60%
I would prefer to avoid an IV unless it is necessary.	46%
I would like to deliver in whatever position is comfortable for me.	72%
I would like to be able to walk around during labor.	81%
I would like to be able to drink fluids during labor.	78%
I would like to be able to eat light foods during labor.	41%
I would like to wear my glasses or contact lenses.	35%
I would like a mirror so I can see the baby's head.	52%

Monitoring

I do not wish to have continuous fetal monitoring unless it is necessary.	32%
I prefer external monitoring to internal monitoring.	60%
I would like continuous fetal monitoring.	39%
I would prefer to be monitored using a fetoscope.	3%
I would prefer to be monitored using Doppler.	12%
I would prefer to be monitored using an external electronic monitor.	22%

Pain Relief

I would like to give birth naturally without medication and use the following methods:	
Bradley Method	9%
Lamaze	28%
Water	
I would like to use a birthing tub for pain relief.	19%
I would like to use a shower for pain relief.	29%
I would like to use massage.	29%
I would like to use acupressure.	4%

I would like to give birth naturally, but would like the following medication to be available should I require it:

Stadol	11%
Nubain	10%
Demerol	21%
Low dose epidural	33%
Epidural block	27%

I would like the following pain relief medication to be administered as soon as possible:

Stadol	6%
Nubain	5%
Demerol	13%
Low dose epidural	16%
Epidural block	26%

INDUCTION

I would like to avoid induction unless there are signs of fetal distress.	65%

Before induction, I would like to try the following natural methods to progress labor:

Relaxation	43%
Herbs	11%
Nipple stimulation	20%

If induction is necessary, I prefer the following methods:

Pitocin	35%
Prostaglandin gel	16%
Amniotomy	7%
Cytotec	3%

EPISIOTOMY

I would prefer to avoid an episiotomy, even if tearing is possible.	21%
I would prefer to avoid an episiotomy unless tearing is possible.	59%
I would like an episiotomy.	7%

DELIVERY OF THE PLACENTA

I would like medication to aid the delivery of the placenta.	25%
I would like to deliver the placenta naturally.	50%
I would like to inspect the placenta after delivery.	14%

CESAREANS

I would like to avoid a cesarean unless it is absolutely necessary.	83%
I would like a second opinion before having a cesarean.	23%
If I have a cesarean, I would like the following anesthesia:	
Epidural	67%
General anesthesia	18%
I would like my partner/coach to be present.	89%
I would like my partner/coach to take photographs.	36%
I would like my partner/coach to video it.	24%
I would like the screen lowered so I can view the birth.	33%
I would like to touch the baby as soon as possible.	81%
I would like my partner/coach to cut the cord.	68%

AFTER THE BIRTH

I would like the baby handed to me immediately after it is born, unless there are signs of fetal distress.	88%
I would like to have the baby evaluated in my presence.	82%
I would like to cut the cord myself.	4%
I would like the umbilical cord to stop pulsating before it is cut.	28%
I have made arrangements to donate the umbilical cord blood.	5%
I have made arrangements to bank the umbilical cord blood.	4%
I would like my partner/coach to cut the cord.	73%
I do not wish to cut the cord.	7%
I would like my baby to be kept with me at all times.	74%

FEEDING

I would like to breast-feed my baby.	65%
I would like to bottle feed my baby.	12%
I will use a combination of breast-feeding and bottle feeding.	21%
Please do not give the baby supplements, pacifiers or glucose solution without consulting me.	67%

IN THE EVENT THE BABY IS SICK

I would like to breast-feed when possible.	78%
I would like unlimited visits for the parents.	86%
I would like to hold the baby when possible.	92%
If it is necessary to transfer the baby to another facility, I would like to follow as soon as possible.	88%

Circumcision

No circumcision is to be performed.	15%
Circumcision can be performed in the hospital.	68%
Anesthesia must be used for the circumcision.	37%
I would like to be present at the circumcision.	25%

Eye Care

I decline eye care for my baby.	4%
I would like to delay eye care until after I have bonded with the baby.	32%
I would prefer erythromycin eye treatment to silver nitrate for my baby.	25%

Vitamin K

I decline vitamin K for my baby.	2%
I would like vitamin K to be administered to my baby.	38%
I would like vitamin K to be given orally.	17%

Birth Plan Worksheet: Your Feelings About the Birth

Describe any fears you have regarding this birth.

    Pain

    Complications

    C-Section

    Length of Labor

    Prematurity

What would help you minimize your anxiety about these issues?

What birth professionals do you feel would best match your birth philosophy and provide the care you desire/need? Why?

    OB

    Family practitioner MD

    Nurse midwife, certified or lay midwife

Doula

Perinatologist

What birth technique most appeals to you?

    The Bradley Method
    Lamaze
    Hypnobirth
    Water birth

What birth location best fits your philosophy and meets your baby's needs?

    Hospital

    Birth Center

    Home

How do you feel about interventions? Which are you willing to consider and which do you strongly wish to avoid?

    IV?
    Induction
    Drugs to induce labor
        Pitocin
        Prostaglandin
    Other methods of inducing
        Stripping/rupturing membranes
        Intercourse
        Nipple stimulation
        Enema/spicy food

Labor Pain
- IV/intramuscular medication
- Regional Anesthesia
    - Epidural
    - Spinal Block
    - Combined Spinal Block/Epidural Block
    - Medications

Fetal monitoring

Operative interventions
- Episiotomy
- Forceps/Vacuum extraction
- C-Section

As you read through this book (don't forget "Birth Around the World"), what appeals to you in terms of ways to make the birth environment as enjoyable as possible and as meaningful as possible keeping in mind the primary goal of a healthy baby?

Who is present?

Who is handling inquiries?

What props?

Birthing positions

Birth balls?

Relaxation techniques

    Methods for coping with labor

    Any special cultural desires

    Handling placenta

    Handling umbilical cord

What are your wishes for your baby's first hour of life?

    Handling of baby

    Umbilical cord

    Placenta

    Repair of your episiotomy

    Bathing

    Eye care

    Vitamins

    Circumcision

    Breast-feeding

Writing Your Birth Plan

Your Birth Plan can be as simple or as complicated as you desire. Include those things that are important to you and your partner. Present it to the others involved with the birth as a wish list and not an ultimatum. Remember to be flexible and be clear that your primary goal is a healthy baby. Try not to be disappointed if things have to be changed, and have some backup plans for an emergency situation, such as a cesarean section or a sick infant.

Also, give yourself the latitude to change your mind during the labor. If you state in your birth plan that you want massage but during labor can't stand it, change your mind! You are the queen during the labor and you don't have to breathe eucalyptus oils or get a massage if you don't want to! No one is going to hold you to it because you thought it sounded nice two months earlier. Same thing with drugs. If you wanted a natural birth but absolutely want pain killers once you are in labor, give yourself latitude to make that decision. Only YOU know (and you may not know until you are in labor) what pain (often referred to by birth practitioners as "discomfort") you can handle and what is too much. If you end up with more pain than you can handle, you may resolutely decide, "I'll NEVER do this again!"

If you would like an e-mail version of the following birth plan, please e-mail the publisher at info@pince-nez.com with the subject line "Sample Birth Plan." Then you will be able to revise it to fit your own situation.

Birth Plan

Dear _____:

My partner and I have created this Birth Plan to help guide all of us in the birth of our baby. I fully understand that we may have to change some of these plans in the interest of a healthy baby. However, it is our hope that we can all work together and make this a happy and healthy birth experience.

Sincerely,

Birth Philosophy

Give a brief introduction of how you feel about birth, how you have prepared for birth, and any particular reservations that you may have. Include reasons why you are giving birth, where you are and why you have chosen a particular birth attendant.

Who will be present (names and roles)

Name those who will attend the birth. Include birth partner, labor support person (list credentials), and any other friends or family members. Do you want them to be present at all times?

First Stage of Labor

- List the prop you want to have: pillows, massage tools, oils, creams, etc.

- Describe the birth environment: lighting, music, etc.

- Do you want to wear your own clothes?

- How do you feel about vaginal exams?

- List any drug intervention you want to have or to avoid having.

- List any drugs you cannot or strongly do not want to be given.

- Do you wish to move about freely?

- List your preferences for moving labor along, if any.

- Discuss the type of fetal monitoring you prefer.

- List the type of hydration you would like: water, ice chips etc.

- If IV prep is necessary, do you prefer a heparin lock?

- Do you want access to a shower or bath tub?

Second Stage of Labor

- Discuss the various positions that you would like to use to assist with labor and delivery.

- State clearly your feelings about an episiotomy. Do you desire perineal massage or any type of compresses?

- If any delivery assistance is necessary, state your preference; e.g., vacuum extraction rather than forceps.

- Do you want to push when you feel the need or when directed by the medical team?

- Do you want to see (by mirror positioning) and feel the head crowning?

- Do you want your partner to "catch the baby"?

- Do you want to wait for the cord to stop pulsing before cutting?

- Do you want your partner to cut the cord?

- Do you want the placenta to deliver naturally or have it medically induced?

First Moments

- Do you want the baby placed on your stomach or chest immediately?

- Do you want to breast-feed immediately?

- State your preference for having newborn tests/procedures performed in the room with you. Also, do you want some to be delayed until the family have had some bonding time?

- Do you want the baby to room-in with you at all times?

- Do you plan to have your partner stay overnight?

- State clearly how you feel about having a pacifier or supplements offered to your baby.

- If the baby is a boy, are you planning to have him circumcised?

- State how long you prefer to stay in the hospital.

- Discuss how you feel about visitors.

Irene's Birth Plan

WHERE

Giving birth in a hospital allows me the opportunity to relax about the birth and focus on the actual process. Getting to the hospital will be the first step of this plan since we need to drive from Napa to San Francisco once labor starts.

LABOR During labor I want to move around as much as possible and have access to a shower. I hope that I will not arrive at the hospital until I am in active labor (cervix dilated 4-7 cms). At that point, I may reques some pain medication. However, unlike my first birth, I may not requst an epidural if the labor progresses quickly. It will depend on my abil ty at the time to handle the pain. The epidural was wonderful last time, particularly for a first birth experience. It felt a little strange, howeve r, to not feel anything and not to know if you are pushing too hard r not enough! Massage and breathing exercises also helped in the early labor last time and I plan to utilize them again. My husband will be my labor coach once again; he did a great job last time! Our labor nurse fr m the last time was wonderful and did so much to help us. My wish is t have another labor nurse just like her. (She is no longer at the hospita —I've checked!)

I would like to suck on ice chips or have a little water to stay hydrated. Hopefully, the hospital will be able to use an external fetal monitor (EFM) or a portable telemetry unit as long as I am walking around.

Delivery

I would like to experiment with positions if I have not received an epidural. Also, I loved having a mirror positioned at the end of the bed last time and watching my daughter being born. I want my husband to cut the cord again and perhaps he can catch the baby at birth this time. Unfortunately not all delivery doctors offer this option.

After Delivery

I want to hold the baby right away and have the opportunity to breast-feed immediately. Last time the hospital staff waited for a while before performing noncritical medical procedures, and this gave my husband and me time to bond with the baby. I plan to keep the baby with me at all times and will go home as soon as I feel able. Having another child to go home to changes things a little! We want her to be a part of her new sibling's life from the very beginning. Last time, staying for two full days at the hospital really helped with breast-feeding and learning how to take care of a brand new little person!!! Hopefully, this time we will not need as much guidance.

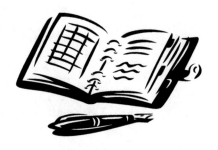

Part Ten: Preparing for the Birth You Have Planned

Prenatal Care

Since this book is about giving birth, it does not go into the prenatal care of you and your baby. Early prenatal care is crucial. This includes nutrition, vitamins, exercise, and possible genetic testing. It means following the baby's growth at regular intervals throughout pregnancy and being aware of possible signs of problems. The average number of prenatal visits is 12 to 14. Consult a birthing professional as soon as you believe you may be pregnant.

The information in this book will help you make decisions about which professionals and environment would best assist you during your pregnancy and help you deliver a healthy baby. By being informed about your options you will have more of a say on how the all important event of the birth of your baby will take place and have the best possible birth experience.

This book also does not go into the care of you and your baby beyond the immediate time after birth. There are many excellent books on postpartum care and recovery available. Read them!

The Prenatal Water Workout

by Jill Cohen

Combining the benefits of water and exercise helps create better births. The women I have worked with tend to have fewer interventions, shorter labors and fewer C-sections. They show fewer complications in the prenatal period and recover faster. The benefits of water are ancient knowledge. While there is no formal documentation of outcomes of labor due to water exercise, I know from three years of observation what is true. It makes perfect sense for the pregnant body to gravitate toward a water environment.

Why water? Exercise in the water is becoming more popular during the prenatal period and offers many benefits for the pregnant mother, both physiological and psychological. Water provides a safe, inspiring atmosphere that women can use and work with as their bodies change and grow.

In order to understand the physiologic dynamic of water, you must understand hydrostatic pressure. When you immerse a body in water up to the shoulders, two great things occur. One is that the body becomes buoyant. The other is that the pressure of water against the skin surface while the body is in motion creates hydrostatic effect, which causes body fluids to move effortlessly upward. For example, if you have swollen feet and you kick through the water, hydrostatic pressure combined with the movement alleviates swelling.

The hydrostatic force of water pushes extravascular fluid into the vascular space, producing an increase in uterine blood flow. Uterine blood flow is essential to grow a healthy baby and placenta. By moving a body immersed to the shoulders and at an adequate depth so that it's not touching the bottom of the pool, hydrostatic pressure makes the blood flow back to the heart more easily. This is an excellent way to stabilize blood pressure.

Another benefit of water workout is alleviation of edema. Movement in water creates twelve pounds of pressure. The pressure squeezes and massages fluid back into the tissue where it is reabsorbed and eliminated. The buoyant effect of a water workout causes no jarring and easier motion, a no-impact form of exercise. The pregnant body can move in ways not possible on land.

Pregnant women should not overheat themselves. Because water has a cooling effect, women can work hard without compromise. Water exercise poses little to no chance of hurting oneself. Buoyancy in pregnancy is so relieving! It enables women to relax and enjoy movement uninhibited.

Jill Cohen has been a lay midwife for 18 years. She is an associate editor at Midwifery Today. Information reprinted with permission of Midwifery Today, Inc.

EXERCISES FOR SECOND STAGE

by Julie Tupler, RN
Editor's Note: While this article as a whole is directed toward the midwife, the exercises are directed toward the pregnant woman and written in language that speaks directly to her.

Women are told to hold their breath and bear down while pushing in labor. The American College of Obstetricians and Gynecologists, in their exercise guidelines, warn women not to do this bearing down maneuver, also called the Valsalva Maneuver, while they are exercising. Recent research also has stated that this can be dangerous, leading to popped blood vessels in the eyes and face, stroke, strain on the supporting ligaments of the bladder and uterus, and also decreased oxygen supply to the baby. So why then are women told to do this in labor? There is one very simple reason: it's easy to do! Anyone can do it. You cannot teach someone a new skill when they are in pain. Exhale pushing with the abdominals is harder to do because it is a new skill and must be learned. However, if this pushing technique is practiced throughout the pregnancy, it becomes second nature in labor. This technique is much more effective, while being easier on the body. A good time to practice this pushing technique is while having a bowel movement.

STRENGTHENING, STRETCHING AND RELAXING THE MUSCLES NEEDED FOR LABOR

It is essential to understand exactly what the abdominal and pelvic floor muscles need to accomplish while pushing in labor in order to understand how to prepare them during pregnancy. I compare pushing in labor to squeezing toothpaste—the tube depicting the uterus and your hand representing the abdominal muscles. When squeezing toothpaste, out of a tube, your hand goes back against the tube of toothpaste and the baby, like toothpaste, comes out the bottom! In order for this to happen, the abdominal muscles must be tight and the pelvic floor muscles must be open and relaxed. Many women in labor, however, make the mistake of simultaneously tightening both the abdominal muscles and pelvic floor muscles. This is like keeping the cap on the toothpaste. Thus it is key to teach women how to isolate and separate these two muscles. This means when they are doing pelvic floor muscle exercises, the abdominal muscles must be relaxed. When they are doing abdominal exercises, the pelvic floor muscles must be relaxed. When they are having a bowel movement, they must think about the abdominals being tight and the pelvic floor muscles being open and relaxed, so that when they get to labor they know how to tighten one and relax the other.

Strong abdominals create the endurance a woman needs for pushing as long as necessary without the muscles fatiguing. A woman also needs to learn how to strengthen, stretch and relax the pelvic floor muscles for labor. Strong pelvic floor muscles are toned muscles, and toned muscles stretch back behind the baby's head instead of going forward with the baby's head. Stretching the muscles with perineal massage prior to delivery will help the stretching process in labor. Learning to relax these muscles, as described above, is key to effective pushing.

Pregnancy Commandment #1: Know Thy Abdominals

Strong abdominals are important to help support the lower spine, improve posture and lessen backaches, as well as for more effective pushing in labor. Four major muscle groups comprise the front abdominal wall:

1. The rectus abdominis is the outermost muscle that runs down the middle of the body from the breastbone to the pubic bone. Its two halves are joined by a fibrous piece of tissue called the linea alba. This muscle may separate (diastasis) during pregnancy due to the pressure of the uterus against it. The rectus abdominis is the support system for the back; and the larger this separation is, the weaker the support system becomes. My exercises will maintain or decrease the size of the diastasis during the pregnancy and will help bring it together after the birth.
2. The external obliques run downward from the rib cage to the pelvis.
3. The internal obliques cross underneath the externals and run diagonally upward from the pelvis to the rib cage.
4. The transverse abdominis is the deepest abdominal muscle and wraps like a corset around the middle. It attaches to the bottom six ribs and the top of the pelvis in the back and wraps around and connects from the linea alba to the recti in the front. The top of the transverse muscle goes behind the recti and the bottom goes in front of the recti.

Both of the obliques, as well as the transverse muscle, attach to the linea alba of the recti. This attachment is very important because the action of one muscle then affects the action of the muscle to which it is attached. We use the transverse abdominis when we breathe, sneeze and cough because the muscle action is forward and backward. This is the muscle we must strengthen for pushing in labor. Because this muscle is attached to the recti muscle, when the transverse goes back towards the spine it brings the recti with it and thus shortens (or strengthens) the recti from the middle of the muscle. It also makes the diastasis of the recti smaller. This principle is the foundation for my "Tupler Technique" abdominal exercises. Conversely, it makes the recti longer (and weaker) and the diastasis bigger. This forward movement applies to a forceful movement such as bearing down—not a passive forward movement used in breathing.

The Tupler Technique

The Tupler Technique involves three exercises using the transverse abdominal muscles. They are the seated transverse, the back-lying pelvic tilt and the headlift.

Seated Transverse

Sit cross-legged on the floor, or in a chair, with your shoulders lined up with your hips. Since the action of the muscle is forward and backward, it works best to imagine the transverse muscle as a sideways elevator with six floors. Use the belly button as the "engine" that moves the muscle forward and backward. First floor is when the transverse is in a relaxed position; fifth floor is when the belly button "touches" the spine; sixth floor is when the belly button goes "out the back" of the spine. The exercise begins by expanding the belly button to the third floor (halfway between the first floor and the fifth floor). This is the starting position of the exercise. The belly button is then pulled back from the third floor to the fifth floor (the spine). Just as in any exercise, in the seated transverse you must squeeze and hold the work part of the exercise, which in this case is the backward movement. Both hands should be placed on the belly, one under the breast on the breastbone and the other on the belly button. The purpose of the hands resting on the abdomen is to make sure that both the top and the bottom of the muscle go in a backward movement. A common mistake that women make is pushing the top part of the muscle forward as the bottom part goes back. You must also count on the backward movement. If you count out loud, it forces you to breathe. The breathing that you are doing during this exercise is shallow chest breathing. If you feel like you are getting out of breath, slow down. Make sure also that you do not have any shoulder or leg involvement when doing this exercise. Besides feeling this exercise in your abdominals, you should feel it in your back. Remember that the transverse is the muscle that wraps around like a corset. The only thing that moves is the belly button.

Do this squeeze and hold movement one hundred times and then rest. This is one set, which should take about two minutes to accomplish. Start with five sets or 500 per day. Do this every day for two weeks. The third week, progress the exercise by now making that backward movement smaller and going from fourth to fifth floor. Continue to do 500 per day. The fourth week, progress to the fifth to sixth (out the back) movement. This is the movement you will be doing for the rest of your pregnancy and until your child is eighteen years old! This fifth to sixth movement is isometric. Do 500 of these for two weeks. In week six, you can wrap a splint (any long piece of fabric) around your waist to bring two halves of the recti together. You pull the splint and maintain this same pull throughout the set of 100. In week seven, you are now ready to start doing ten sets of 100, or 1,000 per day. You should maintain 1,000 or more until the end of your pregnancy.

The larger your abdominals get, the harder this exercise will become. Remember this is really the most important exercise you can do to strengthen your abdominals to prevent back problems during and after pregnancy, as well as prepare them for pushing in labor. With this exercise, you get two for the price of one. Every time the transverse goes back to the spine, it also shortens the recti from the middle of the muscle and makes the diastasis smaller.

Back-lying pelvic tilt

During pregnancy, the abdominals get longer and weaker and the lower back gets shorter and tighter. The purpose of a pelvic tilt is to shorten or strengthen the recti (outermost abdominal muscle) from the bottom of the muscle and lengthen or stretch the lower back.

This exercise is the foundation for the headlift because it covers the first three steps of that exercise. It is important to explain for this back-lying exercise that pregnant women must be cautious about exercising on their backs. I recommend doing this exercise for no longer than three minutes if there are no problems. When the uterus gets larger, it can compress a major blood vessel when a pregnant woman lies on her back. If while lying on her back a woman feels lightheaded or dizzy, this is the first indication that she should roll on her side immediately. This gets the pressure off that blood vessel.

The starting position of this exercise is on the back with heels close to the buttocks, one hand resting on the abdominals and the other hand on your side by the small of your back with your palm facing up. The exercise involves three separate and distinct steps.

<u>Step one</u>: You expand the belly by taking a belly breath.

<u>Step two</u>: You bring "just the belly button" (transverse) to the spine and hold it there. That is why the hand is resting on the belly.

<u>Step three</u>: You think of bringing your pubic bone toward your navel to shorten the recti from the bottom of the muscle, and then you count. Do not use your legs to do this movement. The buttocks do not come

off the floor. This is a small pelvic rock that puts the small of your back on the floor. That is why your hand is by the small of your back.

Do this exercise in sets of twenty and then roll to your side. Work up to three sets of twenty, three times a day.

Headlifts

The purpose of doing a headlift (pregnant or not pregnant) is to shorten or strengthen the recti muscle. The perfect headlift involves shortening the recti from the top, middle and bottom of the muscle. To shorten it from the top, we lift our head. To shorten it from the bottom, we do the back-lying pelvic tilt. These two are automatic and don't really matter unless you shorten the recti also from the middle. To shorten it from the middle, you must use the transverse muscle. There are five things you must know about the transverse muscle to do this exercise correctly.

1. Gravity affects this muscle. It is much harder to work the transverse muscle in a back-lying position. Therefore, we strengthen the transverse muscle in a seated position first so that you acquire the mind/body awareness of a muscle you have never used and also the strength to go out the back (fifth to sixth) as you lift your head and shorten the recti from the middle.

2. The starting position of the muscle is important. We always start this exercise by expanding the belly with a belly breath so the abdominals are in the right starting position to go backwards on the work part of the exercise. Most people inhale while bringing the abdominals back, and then on the exhale lift the head while the abdominals are going forward from the middle.

3. The higher you lift your head, the harder it is to hold the transverse in. If you can't hold the transverse in, then it will go forward and make the middle part of the recti longer. For pregnant women, this would also make the diastasis bigger. So we just barely lift the head. To make the exercise harder, you would bring your heels farther away from your buttocks.

4. The transverse is affected by the way you lift your head. If your head goes straight up (like a turkey imitation), this makes it difficult to hold

the transverse in. This is not a movement we want to accentuate during pregnancy. Therefore, we just lift the head as if we were saying yes (I'm going to get back in those jeans six weeks after delivery!).

5. Counting out loud is important to help you go out the back (fifth to sixth). We recommend that women start headlifts four weeks after starting the seated transverse. At this time they will be doing 500 transverse exercises daily from fifth to sixth floors and will also have mastery of the back-lying pelvic tilt. Prior to that (weeks one to four), a woman can do this five-step exercise without lifting her head. Please remember this is a back-lying position; and if at any time you feel lightheaded or dizzy, roll to your side immediately. The starting position is on the back with the heels close to the buttocks. The hands are now holding the splint. You should be holding the splint with the palms facing down. When you pull the splint you should be pulling the hands toward the belly button. After the pull the hands should be resting on the belly button and breastbone, like in the seated splinted transverse exercises. The purpose is so that you can feel the abdominals working correctly.

<u>Step one</u>: Expand the belly with a belly breath.

<u>Step two</u>: Bring just the belly button (transverse) to the spine (fifth floor) and hold it there.

<u>Step three</u>: Shorten the recti from the bottom with a pelvic rock or shift (this puts the small of your back on the floor).

<u>Step four</u>: Pull the two halves of the splint together.

<u>Step five</u>: (week one through four) Transverse goes out the back (fifth to sixth floor) as you count.

<u>Step six</u>: (week four or when you are doing seated transverse from fifth to sixth floor) Transverse goes out the back (fifth to sixth) as you lift just your head and count. Lift your head as if you were saying yes (I am going to have a great delivery!). Close your eyes to see the transverse working in a backward movement as you lift your head. You may want a friend or partner to put hands on your abdominals when you first start doing this exercise to make sure the abdominals are going in the right direction as you lift your head. Remember, if they go forward instead of backward when you lift your head, you are making the recti

longer from the middle and also making the diastasis bigger. Start with one set of ten headlifts three times per day, then work up to two sets of ten and then three sets of ten. You can then progress to twenty headlifts with the same progress as noted in the ten headlifts instructions.

Using the Transverse with Everything You Do

In the Maternal Fitness™ routine, which can be found in Chapter Eight of *Maternal Fitness* (Simon & Schuster), we use the transverse on the work part of all the exercises. We think of all the power coming from the center. We want you to imagine your transverse lifting your arms when doing the upper body exercises and lifting your head when doing the headlifts. The transverse should be in on the work of any exercise or activity. If you can't hold it in, it is an indication that you need to modify or not do that particular activity or exercise. Don't forget to hold it in when you sneeze, when you cough, when you stand or sit and when you pick up your new baby.

Working the transverse benefits a woman in three important ways:

1. Prevents back problems by maintaining or decreasing the size of the diastasis during the pregnancy and bringing it back together after the pregnancy.

2. Develops an ability for more effective pushing in labor.

3. Promotes faster recovery. If you strengthen this muscle during pregnancy, the muscle will have "muscle memory" and it will be easier to start working this muscle again.

The Kegel Exercise: An Important Exercise or Your Pelvic Floor Future

These muscles that you can't see lie on the floor of the pelvis and figure eight around the urethra (where you urinate), around the vagina and around the recti. They are weakened by the extra weight during pregnancy and by the birthing process. This weakness affects their functions in three ways:

1. Their ability to support the organs in the pelvis decreases. Later in life, you may get a prolapse of organs (your bowel, bladder and uterus may fall).

2. You may get leaking urine when you sneeze or cough.
3. Sexual appreciation may be affected negatively. The walls of the vaginal canal are stretched during birth. Strengthening these muscles will make them long and narrow so something will be felt during intercourse.

It is important to strengthen these muscles not only to help in labor, but also to prevent the problems mentioned above. If a muscle is weak, it will ask another muscle to help it out. The Kegel exercise is therefore done in a seated position with the legs apart (so you don't squeeze your buttock muscles) and your hands resting on the abdominals (so you don't use them while doing this exercise). Close your eyes and pretend you are stopping the flow of urine. Hold that squeeze for ten seconds. At the end of the ten-second hold think of releasing and opening the muscle. This is one repetition. You need to do twenty repetitions (ten-second holds) five times per day. A good time to do them is after doing a set of 100 of the seated transverse exercises, which you are also doing five times per day. If you cannot hold the muscle to ten seconds, start with a five-second hold and work your way up to an eight-second hold and then a ten-second hold. An image that is very helpful in learning how to release and open this muscle is to think of "opening like a little flower." This opening images is very helpful in labor while you are pushing. A good time to practice opening is while having a bowel movement. Remember, your abdominals are back and your pelvic floor is open and relaxed.

Julie Tupler is a Registered Nurse, Certified Childbirth Educator and Trainer, author of Maternal Fitness (Simon & Schuster, 1996), founder of Maternal Fitness™, and advisory board member of Fitness Magazine. For more information on Maternal Fitness, call 212-353-1947 or see her website at www.maternalfitness.com. E-mail: info@maternalfitness.com

Preparing your labor team

LABOR COACH TIPS

While the birth of a baby is a wonderful and sometimes overwhelming experience for the mom, we sometimes forget the effort and energy that is also required from the labor coach. The following tips were collected from partners and coaches who have been there!
- Discuss the birth plan, if there is one, ahead of time.
- Know as much as possible about what is going to happen and what may happen during labor and delivery.
- If you are not sure what is going on at any time, just ask!
- Come prepared with stories, rhymes and other distractions.
- Know and accept that this may be a long process and may not all be under your control.
- Be prepared to be flexible and resourceful.
- Be supportive, no matter what!
- Be an advocate for mom and baby.
- Rest whenever you get the opportunity.

What to bring to the hospital for the new family

So much time goes into preparing for the arrival of the new baby that often the expectant parents do not prepare for their own visit to the hospital or birth center. For a home birth, you do not have to go very far to gather up all that is needed. However, the following lists can be used by anyone awaiting a new arrival. It is always best to plan ahead of time and have everything close at hand, be it in a birth facility or home. There also seems to be something reassuring about having a list in hand!

MOM'S LIST:
- [ ] Birth Plan
- [ ] Nightgown, bathrobe, socks and slippers
- [ ] Hair band and ponytail holder for long hair
- [ ] Face cleanser and moisturizer
- [ ] Body moisturizer and massage oils

- [ ] Lip balm
- [ ] A water spritzer bottle to help keep you cool
- [ ] A camera and film
- [ ] A tape recorder/CD player with batteries (You are not usually allowed to use the electrical outlets at the hospital.)
- [ ] Books, magazines, flowers, candles, photographs, etc.
- [ ] Sanitary napkins
- [ ] Toiletries
- [ ] Nursing bra and breast pads
- [ ] Going-home outfit and comfortable shoes

Birth Partner's List:
- [ ] Snacks
- [ ] A clothing change
- [ ] Overnight toiletry items
- [ ] A book (The laboring mom may very well doze off for a short time.)
- [ ] Cellular phone, phone card or change for the phone
- [ ] Address book with all family and friends' phone numbers

Baby's List:
- [ ] Outfit for the first trip home (include cap and booties)
- [ ] Receiving blanket
- [ ] Diapers
- [ ] Baby nail clippers (most hospitals do not supply then because of liability issues)
- [ ] Infant car seat

What You Will Need at Home

Basics
- [ ] Two packages of disposable diapers (or two dozen cloth)
- [ ] Baby wipes
- [ ] Diaper rash ointment
- [ ] Gentle baby soap
- [ ] No tears shampoo
- [ ] Nasal aspirator
- [ ] 2-4 pacifiers
- [ ] Blunt baby nail scissors

- [ ] Baby brush and comb
- [ ] Alcohol wipes (for the cord and thermometer)
- [ ] Rectal thermometer
- [ ] 4-6 bottles in 4 and 8 ounce size
- [ ] Bottle brush
- [ ] 2 nursing bras (if nursing)
- [ ] Breast pads (if nursing)
- [ ] Breast pump (if nursing)
- [ ] Diaper genie
- [ ] Wipe warmer

CLOTHING
- [ ] 6-8 baby gowns with pull ties
- [ ] 6-8 receiving blankets
- [ ] 4-6 lightweight sleepers
- [ ] 6-8 snap t-shirts or onesies
- [ ] 4 pairs of booties or socks
- [ ] One sweater
- [ ] Snow suit (depending on where you live)
- [ ] 6 bibs
- [ ] 4-6 wash clothes
- [ ] 2-4 hooded bath towels
- [ ] 4 bassinet sheets
- [ ] 2 waterproof mattress pads
- [ ] 3-4 crib sheets
- [ ] 2 quilted crib pads
- [ ] Crib bumper
- [ ] 2 crib blankets (depending on season)
- [ ] 2 comforters (depending on season)

ADDITIONAL ITEMS
- [ ] Infant car seat
- [ ] Crib
- [ ] Bassinet or cradle
- [ ] Baby bathtub
- [ ] Mobile for crib
- [ ] Baby monitor
- [ ] Stroller
- [ ] Baby swing
- [ ] Baby carrier

Part Eleven: Prenatal Fun

A Fun First Day Project: Baby Memory Box

While it is not hard to keep busy after having a baby, it is nice to plan a special project for the "Memory Box" that you can present to your child when she is older. This is a project that a friend of mine told me she and her husband did after their daughter was born.

Collect as many items as possible to place in a box that can be opened when a child reaches a particular milestone. The following are examples of what to include:

- Family photographs.
- Photographs and names of those attending the birth and a "first moments picture."
- That day's newspaper.
- Letters from family and friends welcoming the baby.
- A photograph of the hospital/birth center.
- A photograph of baby's house and nursery.
- A diary of those first few hectic days.
- A list of the current Top Ten books, movies and songs!
- Anything else that is special for the moment!

Belly Casting: Preparation, Creation and Decoration

by Connie Banack, CD

Belly masking (or casting) is a wonderful art form celebrating the amazing transformation of a woman's body during pregnancy. It is usually done two to three weeks before a woman's due date, but can also be used to capture the changes during pregnancy, as well. It is a remarkably simple and inexpensive project, although it's just a little messy! Find out more about this pregnancy art that is rapidly gaining in popularity.

Why would I want to make a belly cast?

A photo captures your body's changes two dimensionally, but a belly cast adds the dramatic third dimension of depth. Although this is a little known way to capture your pregnant body's dimensions, it is also an incredibly wonderful art form. Even if you are uncertain about doing this kind of birth art, do it anyway. As time goes by, and your love for your baby grows, this memento will mean even more to you.

What you will need

- Two to three 8" wide rolls of plaster gauze
- Petroleum jelly
- Plastic wrap for protecting pubic/underarm hair
- Large drop cloth to protect flooring
- Apron or bib for the sculptor
- Chair, bench or low stool
- Bowl, pan or bucket of hot water in which to dip the strips of plaster bandages

Optional:
- Art supplies to decorate body cast, such as plaster of Paris or gesso, if you want to smooth the original rough gauze surface and to enhance features, such as nipples or belly button, as well as strengthen the cast. Also, you might want to use acrylic paints, fabric, yarn, feathers, glitter, beads, dried flowers, photos, etc., for your finishing touches.
- Wire mesh "sandpaper" to get a really smooth plaster surface.
- Shellac, lacquer or glaze to seal and preserve your creation.

Preparation

Sculptor

- Put on old clothes or use an apron and roll up your sleeves. Take off any jewelry.
- Cover the floor with the drop cloth. Make sure the room is warm but well ventilated.
- Assemble supplies and fill the bowl, pan or bucket with warm water.
- Cut the plaster bandages into strips approximately 6, 10 and 14 inches long.
- Generously apply (or have the mother apply) petroleum jelly to the mother's breasts, belly and neck/arms/thighs, anywhere plaster might stick to skin, going no more than half way around her sides and just above the pubic hair. If necessary, use saran wrap or cotton padding to cover armpit, belly or pubic hair. If you don't use enough lubrication, remind the mother to use one of her pain techniques as her hair will be pulled out when the cast comes off!

Mother

Choose your pose. Standing or sitting on the edge of a seat will result in a more round, full-bodied sculpture. Experiment with various poses: lean forward, to one side, back, or against the wall; find the shape/pose you want to preserve. Assume a position in which you can remain fairly still for about 20 minutes to one hour. Don't lie down! This position produces a flattened breast-belly sculpture.

Creation

- Glide one plaster strip at a time through the water for a few seconds. Never let go of the strip, keeping it taut, open and flat (don't let it fold or twist).
- As you pull them up from the water, gently squeeze out the excess water by running your index and middle fingers down the strip.
- Apply the strip to the mother's body. Smoothing and overlapping the strips in various directions strengthens the body cast.
- Work quickly because the plaster begins to set (dry), and the cast begins to separate from her body about 10 to 15 minutes after you begin.
- When you are finished applying the strips (aim for at least two layers of strips), allow the cast to dry for about five minutes, then remove.

Have her help by moving and wiggling to loosen the cast as you gently ease it off at the edges. Once the cast is off, Mom is free to take a refreshing shower! To prevent plaster from clogging up the plumbing, you may want to help wipe the mom down gently with warm washcloths to remove the bits of plaster.

DECORATION

The body cast will need about 24-48 hours to dry completely before you begin decorating it. It may mold if you decide to decorate it before it is done drying.

Before painting or decorating, smooth the surfaces of the cast by applying a thin coat of plaster of Paris or paint it with gesso. For a very smooth finish, sand with the wire mesh.

There is no end to the possibilities: decorate it with paint, a collage of your baby's photos or magazine cutouts, tissue paper designs, dried flowers, beads, feathers, or written messages. After your baby is born, you could even add footprints (right where he/she used to kick you under the ribs) on the sculpture with ink or paint, or make an impression of the footprint in wet plaster on the cast.

Finally, spray or paint with the shellac, lacquer or glaze to finish. If you are doing this yourself, work only in a well-ventilated area, preferably outdoors.

Be creative, and most of all, have fun!

Reprinted with the permission of Connie Banack, a certified doula and childbirth educator residing in Alberta, Canada. She can be contacted at her web site www.mothercare.com.

NOTE:

Web sites selling kits for belly casting indicate that product spec sheets are available. Do not do a belly casting if you are allergic to plaster, petroleum jelly or any other substance that will touch the skin. Do not add anything to the plaster while it is on you that could be toxic! Do all decoration of the plaster cast, including painting, after the cast is off you and only in a well-ventilated area. Avoid using any toxic substances in the decoration of the piece.

Acronyms

When reviewing literature of birth professionals, you will see behind their names just about every possible combination of letters! When you encounter an unfamiliar one, ask what it stands for and which agency, if any, provided that designation. The acronyms may stand for something meaningful (such as a specific education, certification, etc.) or it may be meaningless (except in the eyes of the user!). If it purports to be a certification, research the certifying agency. Ask a birth professional you trust if they have ever heard of them. Find out what that certification involved.

CM	Certified Midwife
CNM	Certified Nurse Midwife
DEM	Direct-Entry Midwife
DO	Doctor of Osteopathy (can be board-certified OB/GYNs)
FACNM	Fellow, American College of Nurse-Midwives
FACOG	Fellow, American College of Obstetricians and Gynecologists
FHT	Fetal heart tones (heart beat)
IVF	In vitro fertilization
OB/GYN	Obstetrician/Gynecologist
VB	Vaginal birth
VBAC	Vaginal birth following a cesarean

Index

Acronyms	218
Apgar	28, 106, 156
Bedrest	160, 170
Belly casting	215
Birth balls	139
Birth customs	171-182
Birthing centers	103, 112
Birth interventions	113
Birth plan	194
Birth plan statistics	184
Birth plan worksheet	189
Birthing positions	135-142
Birth statistics	40
Birthing positions	135
Bradley Method	88
Breast-feeding	48, 160-170
Cesarean sections (C-sections)	27, 38, 43, 46, 54, 121-132
Certified Nurse Midwives/Certified Midwives	58, 73
Childbirth education	82
Circumcision	158
Direct-Entry Midwives (DEM)	58, 74
Doctors of Osteopathic Medicine (DOs)	50
Doulas	33, 76-80
Drugs	115, 116-118
Epidural	19, 21, 23, 28, 32, 117
Episiotomy	119, 157
Eye care of baby	158
Family physicians	51
Fetal monitoring	42, 118
Forceps	120
Gynecologists	51
HIV	122
Heparin locks	114
Herpes	122
Home birth	34, 105, 112
Hospitals	102, 107, 112

Hypnobirth	97
Induction	42, 114, 127
Insurance	52, 53
International Childbirth Education Association	83
IV-Heparin locks	114
Labor	47, 143, 144-152
Labor coach	45, 88, 149, 210, 211
Lamaze	11, 84
Lay midwives	58, 74
OB/GYNs	42, 51
Memory box	214
Midwives	35, 37, 42, 57-76, 94
Nurse midwives	58, 73
Pain medication	25, 116
Perinatologists	51
Physicians	50-56
Pitocin	28, 33, 115
Placenta	156
Prenatal care	41, 61, 200
Postpartum care	62, 159
Prenatal exercises	200-209
Prenatal fun	213
Preparing your labor team	210
Prostaglandin	115
Relaxation and childbirth	143
Spinal block	117
Umbilical cord	155
VBAC	126, 128
Vacuum extraction	120
Vaginal warts	122
Vitamens/Vaccinations	158
Water birth	90-96
What to take to the hospital	210
What you will need at home	211

All Things Considered

In reading the wealth of information sent to me by various organizations and individuals, I feel compelled to include a word or two of caution. All of us, when anticipating the birth of our babies, dream and wish for a speedy labor, an easy delivery and a healthy baby. This is expected. However, we have to remember that while we can stay healthy during pregnancy, arm ourselves with information, and have the best of intentions and plans for our labor and birth, there are times that we will have absolutely no control over events and circumstances. This should not diminish in any way our feelings about the experience of birth or make us feel that in some way we failed or did not do something properly. Please read all these articles carefully and take from each one what best makes sense for you and your birth. Discuss your impressions with your birth professional. Do not become attached to one approach or technique until you have run it by your birth professional to make sure that it will not interfere with the birth of a healthy baby. And remember to be flexible.

There are no right or wrong ways to give birth, just as there are no right or wrong ways to plan for birth. Please prepare for the birth of your baby with one thought at the top of your wish list—a safe birth and healthy baby. Birth is a miracle that comes to all of us in a different way.

Other Parenting Books From Pince-Nez Press

FINDING A NANNY FOR YOUR CHILD IN THE SAN FRANCISCO BAY AREA
by Alyce Desrosiers, LCSW
ISBN: 1-930074-00-X

FINDING A PRESCHOOL FOR YOUR CHILD IN THE SAN FRANCISCO BAY AREA
by Lori Rifkin, Ph.D., Vera Obermeyer, Ph.D., and Irene Byrne, MA
ISBN: 0-9648757-2-1

THE ABC'S OF LEARNING DISABILITIES— FROM A PARENT'S PERSPECTIVE: WHAT YOU NEED TO KNOW TO HELP, UNDERSTAND, AND ADVOCATE FOR YOUR CHILD
by Kim Glenchur, MS, MBA
ISBN: 1-930074-07-7

PRIVATE SCHOOLS OF SAN FRANCISCO & MARIN COUNTIES (K-8)
by Susan Vogel
ISBN: 1-930074-02-6

PRIVATE HIGH SCHOOLS OF THE SAN FRANCISCO BAY AREA
by Susan Vogel
ISBN: 1-930074-08-5

GETTING INTO THE HIGH SCHOOL OF YOUR DREAMS
by Susan Vogel
ISBN: 1-930074-04-2

Order at www.pince-nez.com or call 415-267-5978.